Sexually Transmitted Diseases

A Policymaker's Guide
and Summary of State Laws

D1606946

by

Melissa K. Hough
Prevention Projects Program

and

Julie A. Poppe

National Conference of State Legislatures
William T. Pound, Executive Director

1560 Broadway, Suite 700
Denver, Colorado 80202

444 North Capitol Street, N.W., Suite 515
Washington, D.C. 20001

August 1998

The National Conference of State Legislatures serves the legislators and staffs of the nation's 50 states, its commonwealths, and territories. NCSL is a bipartisan organization with three objectives:

- To improve the quality and effectiveness of state legislatures,
- To foster interstate communication and cooperation,
- To ensure states a strong cohesive voice in the federal system.

The Conference operates from offices in Denver, Colorado, and Washington, D.C.

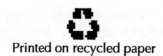

Printed on recycled paper

CONTENTS

List of Tables and Figures

Tables

Figures

PREVENTION PROJECTS PROGRAM

The Prevention Projects Program of the National Conference of State Legislatures (NCSL) works in partnership with the Centers for Disease Control and Prevention to educate state legislators about a variety of public health issues, including HIV and STD prevention, adolescent and school health issues, physical activity, nutrition and tobacco. NCSL's Prevention Projects Program serves state legislatures as an information resource and a forum for communicating with legislative colleagues, experts and government officials around the country.

Legislators and legislative staff of the nation's 50 states, its commonwealths and territories are encouraged to request assistance from NCSL's Prevention Projects Program. The following services are available at no cost to legislators and staff.

www.Stateserv.hpts.org	Meetings and workshops
Information clearinghouse	Presentations to legislative audiences
Publications	Internet database on current year legislation (HIV/AIDS, STDs and adolescent health issues)

Look for the program's home page at www.ncsl.org.

The program is funded through cooperative agreements with the CDC. For further information call Tracey Hooker at NCSL, (303) 830-2200 or e-mail her at tracey.hooker@ncsl.org.

ABOUT THE AUTHORS

Melissa Hough is a policy specialist with NCSL's Prevention Project's Program. Ms. Hough has written publications and articles on various public health issues such as "Sexually Transmitted Diseases and Women;" "Condom Availability in Schools;" *Adolescent Health Issues: State Actions 1992 - 1994*; and *Adolescent Health Issues: State Actions 1995*. She holds a master of social work degree from the University of Denver and a bachelor of social work degree from the University of Wyoming.

Julie Poppe was a private consultant while summarizing the statutes for this publication, but is now at NCSL in the Children and Families Program. She holds a bachelor's degree in social work from the University of Wyoming. Ms. Poppe worked for NCSL's Health Program for two years, then served as a Peace Corps volunteer in Kyrgyzstan.

Preface and Acknowledgments

Sexually Transmitted Diseases: A Policymaker's Guide and Summary of State Laws provides state legislators and legislative staff with an overview of sexually transmitted diseases (STDs) in America today. It is not a medical guide to STDs. Resources in the appendix provide contacts for additional state and federal information that is not included in this publication. The most frequently used acronyms and abbreviations appear on x. Numerous charts and graphs relevant to STDs, state-by-state comparisons, costs and consequences are included throughout the publication as well as in the appendices.

A summary of some 600 STD statutes through 1997 in the 50 states, commonwealths and territories is included.

NCSL appreciates notification of errors and omissions. If you have corrections or requests for further information, please call NCSL's Denver office, (303) 830-2200.

The summaries of any programs or recommendations are not an endorsement by NCSL. This information is merely provided as a broad overview of efforts surrounding the prevention and control of STDs.

Sexually Transmitted Diseases: A Policymaker's Guide and Summary of State Laws was made possible through a cooperative agreement with the U.S. Centers for Disease Control and Prevention (CDC), the National Center for HIV, STD and TB Prevention (NCHSTP), Division of STD Prevention (U87/CCU810205). A special thank you goes to project officer Judy Lipshutz at the CDC's Division of STD Prevention for her continuing support.

NCSL thanks the following reviewers who donated their expertise and time to improving the publication:

- Daniel Daley, Director of Public Policy, Sexuality Information and Education of the United States

- Jennifer Kates, Program Officer, HIV/AIDS Program, Kaiser Family Foundation

- Jacqueline Koenig, Program Officer, Reproductive Health Programs, Kaiser Family Foundation

- Judy Lipshutz, Chief, Planning, Communications and External Relations, Division of STD Prevention, CDC

- Joe McIlhaney, President, The Medical Institute for Sexual Health

- Dennis Murphy, Associate Director, Division of Family and Local Health, New York State Department of Health
- Shepherd Smith, President, The Institute for Youth Development
- Congressman Tom Coburn, U.S. Representative, Oklahoma

The following NCSL staff dedicated many hours to making this publication possible: Tracey Hooker, program director, supervised editing and production; Joanne Stroud, research analyst, provided extensive support for the statute database, and edited and formatted the publication; Stephanie Wilson, staff assistant, compiled some STD statutes, and provided editing and formatting assistance; Julie Poppe, consultant, compiled and summarized the STD statutes; Marie Baca, staff assistant, formatted some of the charts; Lisa Speissegger, CDC public health advisor, and Stephanie Wasserman, policy associate, provided ongoing input and reviewed drafts; Joy Johnson Wilson, committee director, Assembly on Federal Issues Health Committee, NCSL, reviewed the publication; Heather Sidwell, research analyst and Mary Guiden, staff writer from NCSL's D.C. office, reviewed the document; Colleen Moran, University of Denver graduate student intern compiled some STD statutes; Jean East, graduate professor at the University of Denver, provided guidance on the content; Alise Apodaca-Pew, office clerk, input and checked resources; Arturo Perez, senior policy specialist, translated the Puerto Rico statutes; and Leann Stelzer, book editor, edited and supervised production.

West Group provided the list of state STD statute citations.

Thanks to all the unnamed people who provided NCSL with assistance in researching this publication.

The cover design was created by Bruce Holdeman of 601 Design in Denver, Colorado.

EXECUTIVE SUMMARY

Sexually transmitted diseases (STDs) represent a major public health problem in America, where rates are higher than in other industrialized countries. Overall, the estimated economic costs in the United States for selected STDs and related syndromes in 1994 dollars were nearly $10 billion. Both the direct and indirect economic costs associated with disease, combined with quality of life issues for constituents, are compelling reasons for state legislators to address the issue.

STDs are infections that people can contract through sexual contact with someone who is infected. These infections are caused by organisms that live in body fluids like blood, semen and vaginal secretions. They are transmitted via these fluids during vaginal, anal or oral sex. When left untreated or not treated in time, STDs leave lifelong reminders for people, particularly women and children. In large percentages of men and women, symptoms are not evident. Women can become infertile, have a tubal pregnancy or cervical cancer, or live with chronic and severe pelvic pain for the rest of their lives. Infants born to STD-infected mothers suffer from lifelong health problems like brain and neurologic damage that sometimes does not become evident for years. Minorities also are disproportionately affected by STDs, as is the Southern region of the United States. STD rates in these states remain consistently higher than in other states.

This report is designed to provide policymakers with an overview of sexually transmitted diseases. It includes a statute summary of some 600 STD laws that exist in the 50 states, commonwealths and territories through 1997. STDs other than HIV are the primary focus. STD prevention and treatment programs are listed for examples. In addition, state STD project directors and program managers and other resources are included in the appendices, along with the Centers for Disease Control and Prevention National STD Prevention Partnership list.

ACRONYMS AND ABBREVIATIONS

AIDS	Acquired immune deficiency syndrome
CDC	Centers for Disease Control and Prevention
FY	Fiscal year
HB	House bill
HIV	Human immunodeficiency virus (the virus that causes AIDS)
HAV	Hepatitis A virus
HBV	Hepatitis B virus
HCV	Hepatitis C virus
HPV	Human papillomavirus (genital warts)
HSV	Herpes simplex virus
IV	Intravenous or intravenously
IDU	Injecting drug user
OTC	Over-the-counter
PID	Pelvic inflammatory disease
SB	Senate bill
STD	Sexually transmitted disease
STI	Sexually transmitted infection (becoming more commonly used to describe STDs)
TB	Tuberculosis
VD	Venereal disease

1. WHAT ARE STDS?

STDs are an important public health issue for policymakers because of the high costs of health care and the health consequences to their constituents. State policymakers can play a crucial role in STD prevention. They make the decisions about appropriations for services like STD prevention and treatment programs. That yearly amount determines the extent of prevention efforts that are available to stem the spread of STDs in our nation today. Legislators also provide oversight for state government programs and are responsible for bringing issues to the forefront and for making laws that affect the health of constituents.

Sexually transmitted diseases (STDs) infect people of every age, background and socioeconomic level. They are among the most prevalent infectious diseases in the United States, according to the National Institute of Allergy and Infectious Diseases. Although STDs are among the most preventable diseases, more than 12 million cases occur throughout the nation annually; 3 million of those occur in teenagers. Among the 10 most frequently reported diseases in the United States in 1996, five were sexually transmitted— chlamydia, gonorrhea, AIDS, syphilis and Hepatitis B. STDs accounted for 85 percent of all nationally reportable disease cases.[1] See table I and figure I for estimated number of cases of STDs in the United States per year.

Table I. Estimated STD Cases Per Year

Sexually Transmitted Diseases	Estimated Cases per Year
Chlamydia	4 million
Trichomoniasis	3 million
Pelvic Inflammatory Disease	1 million
Gonorrhea	800,000
Human Papillomavirus (Genital Warts)	500,000 - 1 million
Genital Herpes	200,000 - 500,000
Syphilis (infectious)	101,000
HIV	40,000*
AIDS	67,000*
Hepatitis B	53,000
Chancroid	3,500
Congenital Syphilis	3,400
Source: Centers for Disease Control and Prevention, 1995. *Centers for Disease Control and Prevention, 1996.	

Figure 1. Estimated Number of Cases of Selected Infectious Diseases, United States

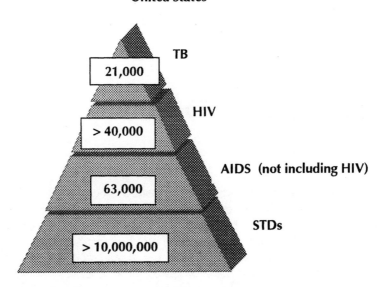

Source: Centers for Disease Control and Prevention, 1996.

Transmission

STDs are infections that people can contract through sexual contact with someone who is infected. These infections are caused by organisms that live in body fluids like blood, semen and vaginal secretions. They are transmitted via these fluids during vaginal, anal or oral sex. Figure 2 demonstrates the basic cycle of transmission.

Some infections, such as genital warts and herpes, are spread by direct skin contact. Hepatitis B and the human immunodeficiency virus (HIV) can be transmitted through intravenous drug injection when needles are shared. Infections can be passed to an infant in the uterus from an STD-infected mother, during birth or through breastfeeding. Transmission to infants occurs in a variety of ways, depending upon the disease. For example, HIV can be transmitted through breastfeeding or in utero, while herpes can be transmitted during delivery if the mother has an active outbreak. The human papillomavirus (HPV) has been detected in the amniotic fluid of pregnant women. [2]

People who have an active case of an STD have a much greater chance of contracting another infection at the same time. In fact, STDs facilitate the transmission of HIV, the virus that causes AIDS. People who have syphilis, herpes, chancroid infection, chlamydia, gonorrhea or trichomaniasis are at three to five times greater risk of acquiring HIV if they are exposed.[3] Likewise, people who have HIV infection and another STD are more likely to transmit HIV than people who have HIV but do not have another STD. Testing for and treating STDs can significantly reduce the spread of HIV infection. For example, a 1995 study in Tanzania, Africa, demonstrated a 42 percent decrease in new, heterosexually transmitted HIV infection in communities where there was greater availability of STD treatment.[4]

Figure 2. Basic Transmission Cycle for STDs

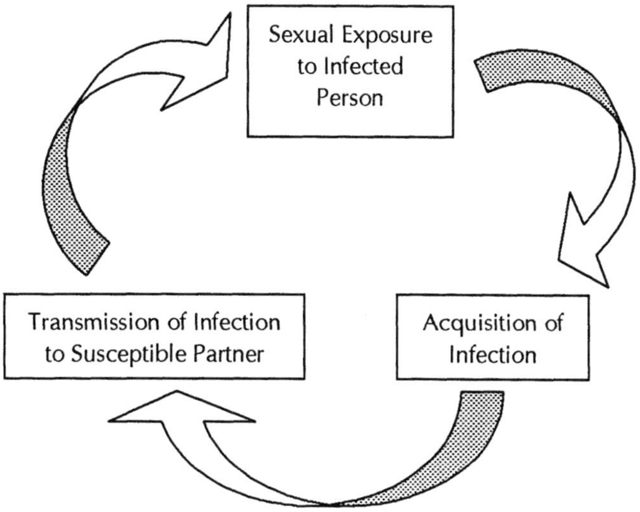

Source: Centers for Disease Control and Prevention, 1996.

Types of STDs

More than 50 infections and syndromes are considered to be sexually transmitted.

There are four types of STDs.

- **Viral** STDs cannot be cured. The most common of these are the human papillomavirus (HPV or genital warts); herpes; Hepatitis A, B, and C; and the human immunodeficiency virus (HIV).

- **Bacterial** STDs can be treated effectively with antibiotics if detected early. The most common bacterial STDs are chlamydia, gonorrhea and syphilis. However, only the infection can be cured—not the damage that already has taken place because the infection was not detected or treated soon enough.

- **Fungal** STDs can be cured. Yeast infection is an example of a fungal disease that can be sexually transmitted.

- **Parasitic** STDs include the more commonly known lice and scabies (mites). They are contracted through close physical contact and are treated with a topical lotion. Trichomaniasis is a parasitic vaginal or penile infection that commonly coexists with other STDs such as gonorrhea. A "flagellated protozoan" is the culprit for infection in trichomaniasis, causing itching, discharge and, sometimes, lower abdominal pain. It can be acquired without direct sexual contact, but that is not typical. It can be cured through treatment with metronidazole (Flagyl, an antibiotic).

Although some STDs were described centuries ago, others have only recently been identified or recognized as being sexually transmitted. Since 1976, eight new diseases have been identified as sexually transmitted (see table 2).

Table 2. Recently Identified Sexually Transmitted Diseases

STD	Year
Human papillomavirus	1976
Human T-cell lymphotropic virus - I	1980
Mobiluncus sp	1980
Mycoplasma genitalium	1981
Human T-cell lymphotropic virus - II	1982
Human immunodeficiency virus - 1	1983
Human immunodeficiency virus - 2	1986
Herpes virus type 8	1995
Source: "Preventing STDs and Pregnancy," *American Medical News.* (February 3, 1997).	

Symptoms

People can be infected with certain sexually transmitted infections and have no symptoms. Some symptoms quickly disappear, leading the infected person to believe that either he or she has no disease or that it went away. Approximately 75 percent of women and 50 percent of men have no symptoms for chlamydia, the most common bacterial STD in the country. If left untreated, 20 percent to 40 percent of women who are infected with chlamydia and 10 percent to 40 percent of women who are infected with gonorrhea develop pelvic inflammatory disease (PID). PID occurs when the disease spreads to the uterus and fallopian tubes. This can lead to infertility, life-threatening tubal pregnancy and severe, chronic pelvic pain. Approximately 100,000 to 150,000 women become infertile each year due to an untreated STD that develops into pelvic inflammatory disease.

When symptoms are apparent, they can range from abnormal genital discharge, burning, painful or difficult urination, lower abdominal pain, odor, swelling or pain in the testicles, itching, blisters or painful open sores, skin rashes, and flu-like symptoms—all depending upon the type of infection. Symptoms also vary from person to person and by gender. Table 3 describes the most common STDs.

Table 3. The Real Facts—The Most Common STDs

STD	New Cases per Year	Curable?	Symptoms	Long-Term Health Effects
Chlamydia	4,000,000	Yes	75 percent of women and 50 percent of men have no symptoms. Symptoms include genital discharge, burning during urination. Women: lower abdominal pain, pain during intercourse. Men: swelling or pain in testicles.	If left untreated, or not treated in time, may lead to pelvic inflammatory disease (PID).
Trichomoniasis or "trich"	3,000,000	Yes	Vaginal discharge, vaginal odor, discomfort during intercourse and painful urination.	Inflammation of fallopian tubes, low birth weight babies and premature infants.
Human Papillomavirus (HPV) or Genital Warts	500,000 - 1,000,000	No	Warts on the vulva, vagina, anus, cervix, penis or scrotum, which may lead to itching, pain or bleeding.	Increased risk of cervical cancer; can be life-threatening.
Gonorrhea	800,000	Yes	30 percent to 80 percent of women have no symptoms. Symptoms include discharge from penis, vagina or rectum and burning or itching during urination. Sore throat.	If left untreated, or not treated in time, may lead to PID and can be life-threatening.
Genital Herpes	200,000 - 500,000	No	Itching or burning in genital area; pain in the legs, buttocks or genital area; vaginal discharge; flu-like symptoms.	Nerve pain; inflammation of spinal cord; urethral strictures; and miscarriage, stillbirth or nonsurviving premature infant.
Syphilis	100,000	Yes	Painless sore (chancre) on genitals or in vagina; skin rash and flu-like symptoms; mild fever, fatigue, sore throat, hair loss and swollen glands throughout body.	In late, or tertiary state, mental illness, blindness, heart disease and death.
Human Immuno-deficiency Virus (HIV)	40,000*	No	Flu-like symptoms, such as fever, loss of appetite and weight, fatigue, and enlarged lymph nodes.	Partial paralysis or weakness of muscles, symptoms affecting the spinal cord, lowered resistance to opportunistic infections, increased risk of cervical cancer, and death.
Pelvic Inflammatory Disease (PID) (A disease resulting from chlamydia or gonorrhea that is left untreated or is not treated in time.)	1,000,000	Yes	Dull to severe pain or tenderness in the lower abdomen, abnormal periods, abnormal vaginal discharge, nausea and/or vomiting, fever and chills.	Damages the fallopian tubes, making it difficult or impossible for a woman to have children. Increased risk for ectopic (tubal) pregnancy, chronic abdominal pain, pelvic adhesions (tissue grows that connects internal organs), pelvic abscesses. Can be life-threatening.

Source: Contraceptive Technology, 1994.
   *Centers for Disease Control and Prevention, 1995 and 1996.

2. WHO IS MOST AFFECTED BY STDS?

Adolescents

Adolescents are at an increased risk for acquiring an STD due to both biological and behavioral factors. In comparison to older women, adolescent and young women are more susceptible to cervical infections such as gonorrhea and chlamydia because the cells of a young woman's cervix is especially vulnerable to infection by certain sexually transmitted organisms.[5]

In addition, youth may be more likely to engage in behaviors that put them at greater risk such as substance abuse, multiple sex partners and unprotected sex. By the 12th grade, nearly 70 percent of students have had sexual intercourse. Approximately 25 percent of these students have had sex with four or more partners (see figure 3).[6]

Figure 3. Percentage of U.S. High School Students Reporting Sexual Activity

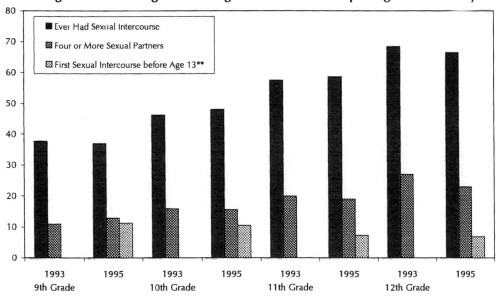

Ever Had Sexual Intercourse
Four or More Sexual Partners
First Sexual Intercourse before Age 13**

**Not reported in 1993

Source: "Youth Risk Behavior Surveillance-United States, 1995," *Morbidity and Mortality Weekly Report*, 45, no. SS-4 (Sept. 27, 1996), U.S. Centers for Disease Control and Prevention.
"Youth Risk Behavior Surveillance-United States, 1995," *Morbidity and Mortality Weekly Report*, 44, no. SS-1 (March 24, 1995), U.S. Centers for Disease Control and Prevention.

The American Social Health Association (ASHA) reports that 52 percent of teenagers get most of their information regarding STDs from school. Twenty-five percent of teens get their information from books, magazines and TV; 11 percent get it from parents and other family members; 7 percent get their information from other sources; and 5 percent get it from their health care providers.[7]

Adolescents also may not have adequate access to STD-related services, or, if they do, they may not take advantage of the care that is available. Barriers to gaining access to STD services for adolescents include lack of insurance or other ability to pay, lack of transportation, discomfort with facilities, services that are designed for adults, and concerns about confidentiality.[8] One of every four adolescents and young adults does not have health insurance coverage. Figure 4 illustrates the distribution of 15 to 29 year olds in the United States by health insurance coverage.

Figure 4. Distribution of 15- to 29-Year-Old People in the United States By Health Insurance Coverage, 1993

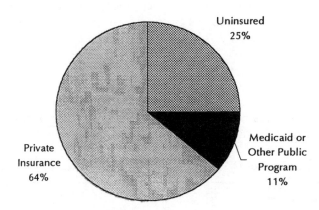

Source: UCLA Center for Health Policy Research, unpublished data, 1996.

Women

Due to anatomical differences, women are more at risk of acquiring an STD than men. After one act of unprotected intercourse with an infected partner, a woman is more likely to be infected with gonorrhea, chlamydia, HIV or Hepatitis B than a man. In addition, STDs that are left untreated can lead to greater complications in women, including pelvic inflammatory disease (PID), tubal pregnancy, chronic pain and infertility.

Some STDs are associated with cancers of the cervix, vagina, vulva, anus and penis. These cancers are strongly associated with certain types of human papillomavirus infection. Between 60 percent and 90 percent of genital cancers are HPV-associated.[9] Cervical cancer is the second leading cause of cancer deaths in women worldwide, and the most common cause of STD-related death (see figure 5).[10]

A 1994 study of 1,000 women, however, found that 84 percent of those surveyed do not think they are at risk of contracting STDs. Even those in high-risk groups—women under age 25 or those who have had multiple sex partners—are unaware of their risks.[11]

Figure 5. Causes of STD-Related Deaths Among U.S. Women, 1992

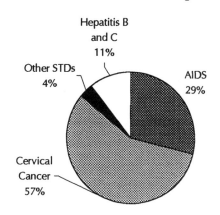

Source: Ebrahim S.H., Peterman T.A., Zaidi A.A., Kamb M.L. "Mortality Related to Sexually Transmitted Diseases in Women, U.S., 1973-1992." *Proceedings of the Eleventh Meeting of the International Society for STD Research,* August 27-30, 1995, New Orleans, La.

Many women also are not adequately screened for STDs, according to a recent survey conducted by the Kaiser Family Foundation and *Glamour* magazine.[12] The study found that only 12 percent of the 482 women surveyed between the ages of 18 and 44 reported that their health provider brought up the issue of sexually transmitted disease during the first exam.   Women surveyed had been to a new provider during the past year for routine gynecological and obstetrical care.   More often than not, the patient's medical history is discussed during that first visit.   Sixty-four percent of the women felt it was up to the provider to initiate conversation about STDs.   Only 3 percent of women surveyed initiated the conversation with the provider themselves (see table 4 for survey results).   As part of a "routine assessment," the American College of Obstetrics and Gynecology (ACOG), in its *Guidelines for Women's Health Care,* recommends evaluation and counseling about STDs for all women under age 65.

Table 4. Percent of Women Who Said Topic Discussed During First Visit With New Doctor or Health Professional for Gynecological or Obstetrical Care

Topic	Topic raised by the health professional	Topic raised by the patient	Topic raised at the first visit *
Breast Self Exam	69%	4%	74%
Pap Smear	60%	12%	74%
Birth Control	33%	20%	54%
Mammograms	34%	7%	41%
Sexual History and/or Current Sexual Activity	36%	3%	39%
Alcohol Use	24%	1%	25%
HIV/AIDS	19%	2%	21%
STDs other than HIV/AIDS	12%	3%	15%
* Percentages in the first two columns may not add up to the percentages in the third column because of rounding or respondents answering "Don't know" to the question "Who initiated this conversation?"			
Source: Kaiser Family Foundation/*Glamour* National Survey on STDs, 1997.			

Pregnant Women

A pregnant woman is at risk for the same consequences of STDs as a woman who is not pregnant, including cervical and other cancers, chronic Hepatitis, cirrhosis and other complications.[13] However, pregnant women may suffer double consequences: not only is the mother at risk, but so is her unborn child. During pregnancy, some of the consequences a woman may experience are early labor, premature rupture of the membranes surrounding the baby in the uterus, and uterine infection after delivery.

STDs can be passed from mother to infant before, during or after birth. Syphilis crosses the placenta and infects the fetus during development. Gonorrhea, chlamydia, Hepatitis B and C, and genital herpes are transmitted from mother to infant as the infant moves through the birth canal. HIV can be transmitted to an infant through the placenta during pregnancy, during birth, and through breast milk.[14] Table 5 shows the annual estimated number of pregnant women in the United States who have specific STDs.

Table 5. Estimated Number of Pregnant Women in the United States Per Year with Specific STDs

STDs	Estimated Number of Pregnant Women
Bacterial Vaginosis	800,000
Herpes Simplex	800,000
Chlamydia	200,000
Trichomaniasis	80,000
Gonorrhea	40,000
Hepatitis B	40,000
HIV	8,000
Syphilis	8,000

Source: R.L. Goldberg et al., "Sexually transmitted diseases and adverse outcomes of pregnancy," *Clinics in Perinatology: Infections in Perinatology* 24, no. 1 (1997): 23-41.

Infants

With the increase in sexually transmitted infections, adverse pregnancy outcomes have increased in America in recent years. Preventing STDs is one important way to decrease many serious health problems in newborns.

The effects of STDs on newborns may appear at birth or may not be detected for months or even years. STDs can have many harmful effects on newborns. They include stillbirth, low birth weight, eye infection (conjunctivitis), pneumonia, blood stream infection (neonatal sepsis), brain damage or motor disorder (neurologic damage), congenital abnormalities such as blindness, deafness or other organ damage, acute Hepatitis, meningitis, chronic liver disease and cirrhosis.[15]

In 1993, more than 3,000 babies were born with syphilis. Fetal or newborn death occurs for up to 40 percent of babies born to mothers who have untreated syphilis. At least 40 percent of infants born alive to mothers who have untreated early syphilis may suffer from brain damage, blindness and serious bone deformities. Pregnant women who are infected with chlamydia or gonorrhea have been shown to be at increased risk for postpartum endometriosis—a condition where uterine lining tissue is in places other than the uterus, causing extreme pain and other health problems. Twenty percent to 50 percent of infants who are born to women infected with chlamydia develop eye infections, and 10 percent to 20 percent develop pneumonia.

Effects on infants can be avoided through STD prevention and treatment before and during pregnancy. The CDC *STD Treatment Guidelines* recommend that pregnant women be screened for chlamydia, gonorrhea, Hepatitis B, HIV and syphilis. Antibiotics can treat and cure bacterial STDs like chlamydia, gonorrhea and syphilis during pregnancy. However, viral STDs like HIV and genital herpes cannot be cured. Only the symptoms may be reduced with antiviral medication.[16] Treatment of the mother with zidovudine (AZT) for HIV during pregnancy can reduce HIV infection rates in infants by approximately 66 percent.[17] (The state statute summary in chapter 8 includes laws that relate to prenatal and postnatal testing for STDs.)

Minorities

When compared with rates for whites, surveillance data reported higher rates of STDs for some racial or ethnic groups. African-Americans and Hispanic Americans, for example, have higher reported rates of chlamydia, gonorrhea and syphilis than do European Americans.[18] In 1996, for example, the gonorrhea rates for African-Americans were 32 times greater than those of whites; gonorrhea rates for Hispanics were almost three times greater than those of whites. Surveillance data may be biased because minority populations are more likely to use public clinics where reporting is more common than among private or other providers.

In the United States, race and ethnicity are markers that correlate with other, more fundamental, determinants of health status. These determinants include poverty, access to quality health care, health care seeking behavior, illicit drug use and living in communities where there is a high prevalence of STDs. The CDC believes that one of the first steps toward empowering communities to organize and focus on this problem is to acknowledge the difference in STD rates among racial and ethnic groups.[19]

Geographic Distribution

STDs disproportionately affect people who live in the Southern states (Alabama, Arkansas, Delaware, Florida, Georgia, Kentucky, Louisiana, Maryland, Mississippi, North Carolina, Oklahoma, South Carolina, Tennessee, Virginia and West Virginia and the District of Columbia). The Southern region consistently has higher rates of primary and secondary syphilis and gonorrhea than any other region throughout the 1980s and 1990s. Similar trends have been seen in the South for chlamydia, although widespread reporting has begun only recently and remains incomplete in many states. Six of the 10 states with the highest rates of chlamydia were in the South. Ten of the states with the highest rate of gonorrhea were Southern states, and eight of the 10 states with high rates of primary and secondary syphilis were in the South. The reasons for these higher rates are not clear, but may include differences in racial and ethnic distribution of the population, poverty, and availability and quality of health care services.[20] Tables 6, 7 and 8 and figures 6, 7 and 8 provide additional STD statistics by state.

**Table 6. Chlamydia—Reported Cases and Rates by State/Area,
Ranked According to Rates, United States and Outlying Areas, 1996**

Rank	State/Area	Rate per 100,000
	U.S. Total[1]	194.5
1	New York[2]	361.8
2	Delaware	316.6
3	South Carolina	255.7
4	Louisiana	253.8
5	Arizona	253.5
6	Tennessee	249.7
7	New Mexico	237.7
8	Maryland	236.0
9	Texas	229.7
10	Alaska	225.3
11	Oklahoma	225.1
12	Missouri	224.7
13	Guam	215.4
14	South Dakota	211.0
15	North Carolina	209.6
16	Michigan	208.0
17	Illinois	206.5
18	Wisconsin	200.9
19	Alabama	195.3
20	California	194.9
21	Colorado	194.4
22	Connecticut	191.4
23	Georgia	188.2
24	Nevada	186.1
25	Ohio	185.2
26	Rhode Island	185.2
27	Indiana	178.1
28	Virginia	177.6
29	Kentucky	176.3
30	Florida	174.8
31	Oregon	173.8
32	Kansas	173.4
33	Washington	170.1
34	Mississippi	161.3
35	Pennsylvania	159.7
36	North Dakota	158.4
37	New Jersey	154.5
38	Hawaii	153.0
39	Nebraska	151.4
40	Iowa	146.6
41	Idaho	131.0
42	Wyoming	129.3
43	Montana	129.2
44	West Virginia	127.2
45	Minnesota	121.6
46	Massachusetts	112.6
47	Arkansas	85.0
48	Utah	81.9
49	Maine	77.9
50	Vermont	68.1
51	Puerto Rico	66.7
52	New Hampshire	63.8
53	Virgin Islands	9.9

1. Includes cases reported by Washington, D.C., but excludes Guam, Puerto Rico and the Virgin Islands.
2. New York's rate is based on New York City. No cases were reported outside New York City.
Source: Centers for Disease Control and Prevention, 1997.

Figure 6. Chlamydia
Rates by States, United States and Outlying Areas, 1996

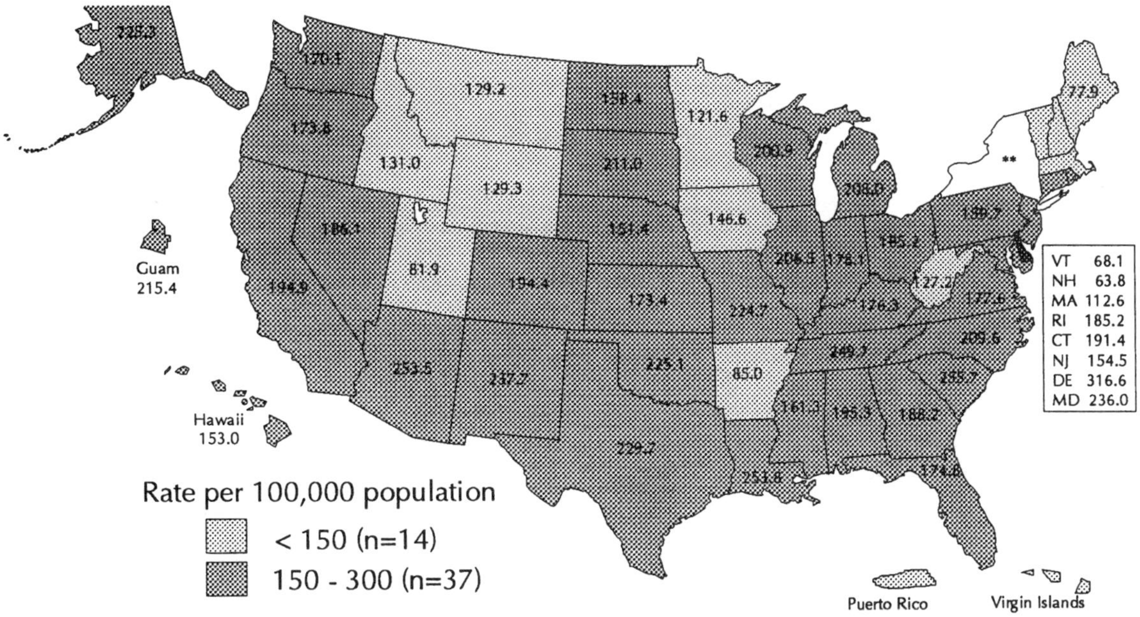

VT	68.1
NH	63.8
MA	112.6
RI	185.2
CT	191.4
NJ	154.5
DE	316.6
MD	236.0

Guam
215.4

Hawaii
153.0

Rate per 100,000 population

< 150 (n=14)

150 - 300 (n=37)

Puerto Rico   Virgin Islands

Notes: The rate of chlamydia for the United States and outlying areas (including Guam, Puerto Rico and the Virgin Islands) was 192.6 per 100,000 population.
**The New York City Rate was 361,8 per 100,000 population. No cases were reported outside New York City.

Source: Centers for Disease Control and Prevention, 1997.

**Table 7. Gonorrhea—Reported Cases and Rates by State/Area,
Ranked According to Rates, United States and Outlying Areas, 1996**

Rank	State/Area	Rate per 100,000
	U.S. Total[1]	124.0
1	South Carolina	317.5
2	Alabama	309.6
3	Georgia	275.1
4	North Carolina	253.4
5	Mississippi	250.0
6	Maryland	229.9
7	Tennessee	222.8
8	Louisiana	214.5
9	Arkansas	203.6
10	Delaware	203.0
11	Michigan	158.4
12	Missouri	158.2
13	Illinois	151.9
14	Oklahoma	149.4
15	Virginia	140.4
16	Florida	135.4
17	Ohio	134.0
18	Texas	123.5
19	Indiana	114.4
20	New York	113.6
21	New Jersey	109.8
22	Kentucky	109.6
23	Connecticut	103.5
24	Pennsylvania	89.5
25	Arizona	87.9
26	Wisconsin	87.5
27	Kansas	79.7
28	Alaska	77.2
29	Nebraska	71.1
30	Nevada	67.0
31	California	59.0
32	Minnesota	58.5
33	New Mexico	52.8
34	Rhode Island	49.1
35	Hawaii	41.9
36	Iowa	40.3
37	West Virginia	40.3
38	Guam	39.7
39	Washington	37.2
40	Colorado	36.5
41	Massachusetts	36.0
42	Oregon	28.2
43	South Dakota	24.1
44	Puerto Rico	17.4
45	Utah	14.2
46	New Hampshire	13.3
47	Virgin Islands	10.8
48	Wyoming	8.5
49	Idaho	8.4
50	Vermont	8.0
51	North Dakota	5.8
52	Maine	4.4
53	Montana	4.4

1. Includes cases reported by Washington, D.C., but excludes Guam, Puerto Rico and the Virgin Islands.

Source: Centers for Disease Control and Prevention, 1997.

Figure 7. Gonorrhea
Rates by State, United States and Outlying Areas, 1996

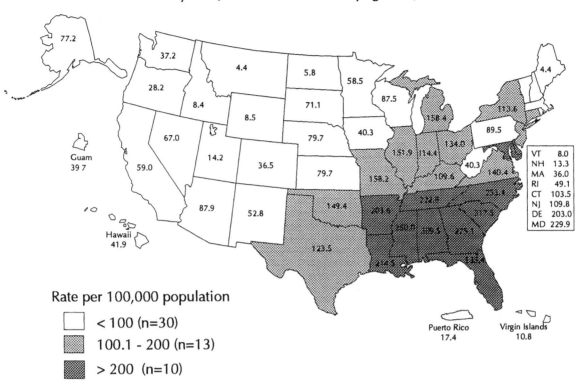

Rate per 100,000 population

- ☐ < 100 (n=30)
- ▨ 100.1 - 200 (n=13)
- ▦ > 200 (n=10)

VT	8.0
NH	13.3
MA	36.0
RI	49.1
CT	103.5
NJ	109.8
DE	203.0
MD	229.9

Note: The rate of gonorrhea for the United States and outlying areas (including Guam, Puerto Rico and the Virgin Islands) was 122.4 per 100,000 population. The Healthy People 2000 objective is 100 per 100,000 population.

Source: Centers for Disease Control and Prevention, 1997.

Table 8. Primary and Secondary Syphilis—Reported Cases and Rates by State/Area, Ranked According to Rates, United States and Outlying Areas, 1996

Rank	State/Area	Rate per 100,000
	U.S. Total[1]	4.3
1	Mississippi	30.4
2	Tennessee	16.2
3	North Carolina	14.6
4	Maryland	14.5
5	Alabama	12.4
6	Louisiana	12.3
7	South Carolina	10.9
8	Arkansas	10.5
9	Virgin Islands	9.9
10	Georgia	9.6
11	Virginia	5.9
12	Puerto Rico	5.6
13	Oklahoma	5.5
14	Ohio	5.2
15	Delaware	4.9
16	Texas	4.8
17	Illinois	4.2
18	Missouri	4.2
19	Kentucky	4.0
20	Indiana	3.6
21	Wisconsin	3.4
22	Connecticut	3.1
23	Florida	2.6
24	Arizona	2.4
25	New Jersey	2.2
26	Michigan	1.9
27	California	1.6
28	Massachusetts	1.4
29	Pennsylvania	1.4
30	Nevada	1.3
31	New York	1.2
32	Kansas	1.1
33	Iowa	0.8
34	Colorado	0.7
35	Wyoming	0.4
36	Rhode Island	0.4
37	West Virginia	0.4
38	Nebraska	0.4
39	Minnesota	0.3
40	Idaho	0.3
41	Oregon	0.3
42	Hawaii	0.3
43	New Mexico	0.2
44	Washington	0.2
45	Utah	0.2
46	New Hampshire	0.1
47	Maine	0.1
48	Alaska	0.0
49	Montana	0.0
50	North Dakota	0.0
51	South Dakota	0.0
52	Vermont	0.0
53	Guam	0.0

1. Includes cases reported by Washington, D.C., but excludes Guam, Puerto Rico and the Virgin Islands.

Source: Centers for Disease Control and Prevention, 1997.

Figure 8: Primary and Secondary Syphilis Rates by State, Unites States and Outlying Areas, 1996

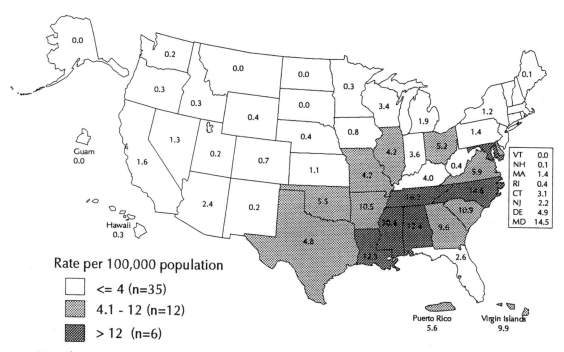

Rate per 100,000 population

☐	<= 4 (n=35)
▒	4.1 - 12 (n=12)
▓	> 12 (n=6)

VT	0.0
NH	0.1
MA	1.4
RI	0.4
CT	3.1
NJ	2.2
DE	4.9
MD	14.5

Note: The rate of primary and secondary syphilis for the United States and outlying areas (including Guam, Puerto Rico and the Virgin Islands) was 4.4 per 100,000 population. The Healthy People 2000 objective is 4.0 per 100,000 population.

Source: Centers for Disease Control and Prevention, 1997.

3. WHY IS THIS ISSUE IMPORTANT FOR POLICYMAKERS?

STDs are costly. Overall, the estimated total costs (see box) for selected STDs and related syndromes in 1994 dollars were nearly $10 billion.[21] This rough estimate includes the most prevalent STDs, but does not include such STDs and syndromes as vaginal bacteriosis, trichomaniasis, scabies and others. This estimate also does not include the cost of sexually transmitted HIV infections, which is estimated to be at least $6.7 billion. It also does not include the cost of premature births that result from STDs. When HIV costs are added to the total of STD-related costs, the costs increase to a total of nearly $17 billion. These numbers represent the tremendous need in America for effective STD prevention programs (see table 9).

STD Costs

When estimating the economic affects of STDs on society, both direct and indirect costs are considered. *Direct costs* mean the expenditures for health care and represent the value of goods and services that were actually used to treat STDs or their associated consequences. They include medical or non-medical services and materials such as costs for health professionals, services, laboratory services, hospitalizations for an STD-related condition, transportation, residential care and special education programs (e.g., for children who suffer lifelong consequences as a result of in vitro STD infection).

Indirect costs refer to lost productivity and represent the value of output foregone by individuals who have STDs and associated disabilities. These costs include lost wages because of not working due to STD-related illness. Premature death also is calculated into the indirect costs of STDs.[22]

In order to determine the costs associated with STDs, the Institute of Medicine's Committee on Prevention and Control of STDs commissioned a paper to provide a basis for the estimations.[23] One of the major challenges to estimating costs is the lack of uniformity and consistency in nationwide STD reporting. Each state has the authority to determine which diseases or health conditions are to be reported to health departments by practitioners. Syphilis and gonorrhea are reportable diseases in all 50 states. New York currently is the only state that does not require chlamydia reporting. Nevertheless, these common STDs often are underreported. One reason for underreporting is that providers, particularly in the private sector, simply do not report.[24] In addition, the people who never seek treatment for disease or do not know they are infected are not accounted for in these estimates.

Table 9. Estimated Costs of Selected STDs and Resulting Conditions
United States, 1994
(1994 dollars, in millions)

STDs	Direct Cost	Total Cost
Pelvic Inflammatory Disease (PID)	$3,119.0	$4,148.0
Human Papillomavirus (HPV)	2,878.0	3,828.0
Chlamydia	1,514.0	2,014.0
Gonorrhea	791.0	1,052.0
Cervical Cancer*	554.0	737.0
Hepatitis B Virus (HBV)	117.0	156.0
Herpes	178.0	237.0
Syphilis	79.0	106.0
Chancroid	0.7	0.9
Subtotal STDs (excluding HIV/AIDS)	**$7,484.0**	**$9,954.0**
Sexually Transmitted HIV	$5,025.0	$6,683.0
Total (including HIV)	**$12,509.0**	**$16,638.0**

Source: Institute of Medicine, 1996.
* Estimate assumes 70 percent of cervical cancer is STD-related.

Figure 9. Estimated Total Costs Associated with STDs (excluding HIV)
Compared to the National Public Investment in STD Prevention for 1994

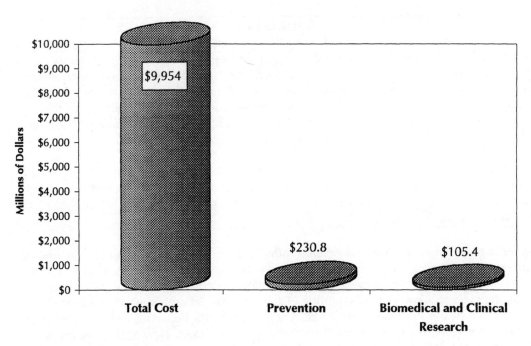

Source: Institute of Medicine, 1996.

Sexually transmitted diseases represent a major public health problem in America, where rates are higher than in other industrialized countries. Both the direct and indirect economic costs associated with disease, combined with quality of life issues for

20

constituents, are compelling reasons to address the issue. Yet, raising the issue generally is difficult. It is difficult for some people to talk about sex in the privacy of their own homes, let alone on the senate floor. In fact, public health workers who specialize in STD prevention, control and treatment are trained for many months until they can discuss sex and STDs with patients. It is understandable, then, that it would be a challenging issue to bring before the legislature. Given the tremendous effects of STDs on society— more than 12 million cases nationwide—the problem merits state legislative attention.

4. Funding and Provision of Services

Who pays for STD-associated expenses? Data are limited, but a study from 1983 through 1987 of payment sources for pelvic inflammatory disease found that public payment and private insurance sources covered 30 percent and 41 percent, respectively, of the direct costs.[25]

STD prevention and treatment activities in the United States consist of both public and private efforts. Activities include the delivery of services by health care providers; disease monitoring and tracking; information systems; training and education of health care professionals; and funding of education, prevention and treatment programs. Most programs are publicly sponsored. Some programs, such as training and education of health professionals, are supported by both the public and private sectors. National health surveys are directed and carried out by the federal government, and disease monitoring and tracking takes place at all levels of government and throughout the private sector.[26]

Clinical services for STDs include screening, diagnosis and treatment, patient counseling, partner notification and treatment. These services are provided primarily in three types of settings—dedicated public STD clinics, community-based health clinics, and private health care settings.[27]

Dedicated public STD clinics refer to publicly funded clinics that mainly provide STD-related services, specifically diagnosis and treatment, and notification of exposed partners. Dedicated public STD clinics are located in every state, every major city, and most counties and small cities in the United States. They were established on the premise that most people who have STDs prefer anonymous and confidential services, are not able to afford care at other clinics, or simply are unable to obtain care from private sector professionals because these professionals are unable or unwilling to provide STD-related care. These clinics provide services to a large number of patients. Most charge only a nominal fee or have a sliding fee scale for services. The client base is disproportionately male. Patients who visit public STD clinics typically have symptoms of infection and other health problems such as HIV infection, unintended pregnancy, and drug and alcohol use.[28]

Funding for the clinics include a combination of federal, state and local funds. The only federal agency that supports dedicated public STD clinics is the Centers for Disease Control and Prevention (CDC). The CDC primarily funds prevention services such as patient education, partner notification and outreach, rather than direct clinical services. Most financial support for the clinics comes from state and local health departments.

A significant proportion of the patients who obtain services at dedicated public STD clinics have private insurance coverage (see Figure 11). A 1995 survey found that approximately 31 percent of male and 24 percent of female patients seen in dedicated public STD clinics had private insurance.[29] One explanation for these numbers is that adolescents go to the dedicated public STD clinics for services because of confidentiality. Here they do not have to report to the insurance company that they were seeking treatment for STDs. Thus, the health departments pay these costs for people who already are insured privately.[30]

**Figure 10. Distribution of Health Insurance Status
Among People Using Public STD Clinics, 1995**

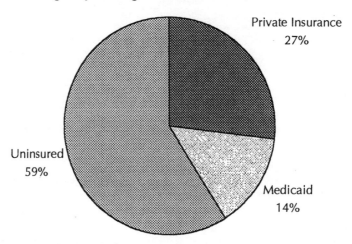

Source: Celum C.L., et al. "Where would clients seek care for STD services under health care reform? Results of a STD client survey from five clinics." Eleventh Meeting of the International Society for STD Research, August 27-30 1995, New Orleans, La.

Community-based health clinics include family planning clinics, prenatal clinics, youth and teen clinics, homeless programs, community-based health centers, and school-based clinics. Similar to the dedicated public clinics, community-based clinics see a high volume of patients and provide care at low or no cost to the patient. STDs are not the primary focus of these clinics, but STD services are provided along with other health care services. Clients tend to be younger, from lower socioeconomic class communities and of certain ethnic and racial groups. More women and children use the clinics than men.

The major difference between dedicated public STD clinics and community-based health clinics is that people depend on community-based health clinics for regular health care, unlike the dedicated clinics where people go specifically for STD diagnosis and treatment. In addition, STDs identified at the community-based health center are more likely to be found through screening rather than through symptoms of disease.[31]

Private health care settings like private physician offices, private clinics and private hospital emergency rooms provide some STD services. One complication in the private setting for managing STDs has to do with the treatment guidelines, which are not used in private settings to the extent they should be. Due to underreporting in private health care settings, data is limited about the number of STD cases identified and the costs and expenditures related to diagnosis and treatment of STDs.[32]

In addition to the previous sources for STD services, such sources also can be provided to school-age youth and university students through *school- and university-based centers.* These health centers strive to provide accessible, appropriate, affordable and effective health care in a setting aimed specifically at young people. They provide primary health care services in addition to STD-related services. Although school-based health centers are found in 45 states and the District of Columbia, only 12 percent of school districts in the United States have at least one school-based or school-linked clinic.[33, 34]

Where do people actually go for STD treatment? Data are limited, but a 1997 study found that 59 percent of patients went to a private provider for services, and 15 percent went to clinics other than an emergency room, public STD clinic or family planning clinic. Ten percent went to the emergency room, 9 percent went to an STD clinic, and 7 percent went to a family planning clinic for services.[35]

5. FEDERAL ACTIVITY

The federal government has played a role in controlling the spread of STDs since the early part of the 20th century.[36] The National Venereal Disease Control Act, passed in 1938, established the federal program for states to conduct screening and other activities through grants.[37] Section 318 of the Public Health Service Act authorizes the Department of Health and Human Services (DHHS) to make grants and assist states, their political subdivisions, and public and nonprofit private entities in STD prevention and control, research, demonstration programs, and provide public information and education programs. DHHS is authorized to provide training, education and clinical skill improvement for health-care providers.[38]

Publicly funded STD programs have been remarkably successful for certain STDs, according to the Centers for Disease Control and Prevention. Aggressive national syphilis programs initiated in the late 1940s and early 1950s nearly eradicated syphilis in the United States. However, it is important to note that syphilis treatment was not successful in some minority communities. Cases continued to decline through 1956, when they reached an all-time low of 3.9 cases per 100,000 people. An assumption was made that the problem was solved, resulting in a sharp decline in funding. Within four years, the incidence of primary and secondary syphilis nearly tripled. Syphilis cases continued to increase until 1990, when the rate reached 20.3 cases per 100,000 people. Since that time, syphilis has decreased, nearing the 1956 rate. The CDC is launching a syphilis elimination effort, but this will require increased resources to ensure long-term success.[39]

National programs to combat gonorrhea were initiated in the early 1970s and continued through the early 1980s. National cases dropped 59 percent from 1978 to 1994. The rate of gonorrhea has continued its overall decline since 1974. The rate decreased 17 percent, from 149.4 cases per 100,000 people in 1995 to 124 per 100,000 people in 1996.[40]

The Preventive Health Amendments of 1992 modified Section 318 of the Public Health Service Act and authorized the CDC to implement screening and treatment programs for STDs that cause infertility in women. In addition, the amendments authorized grants to conduct research to determine methods to improve the delivery of STD-related infertility prevention services. The responsibility for carrying out this congressional mandate was assigned to the CDC's Division of STD Prevention.

The federal fiscal year 1998 budget included an increase of $7.5 million for the Centers for Disease Control and Prevention's Infertility Program. This was the only increase in the $106 million CDC budget for STDs. (Figure 11 and table 10 show congressional appropriations for 20 years of CDC STD programs.) In addition, the president's budget asked for a 3 percent increase for the National Institutes of Health to be used for STD research. The National Institute of Allergy and Infectious Diseases received a 4 percent increase, the largest for any of the institutes.[41]

Professionals in the STD field argue that federal funding has not kept up with the growing STD problem or today's dollars (see figure 11). History has demonstrated that STD cases rise as funding declines and, as funding rises, cases decline.

Figure 11. Congressional Appropriations for CDC STD Programs Since 1975

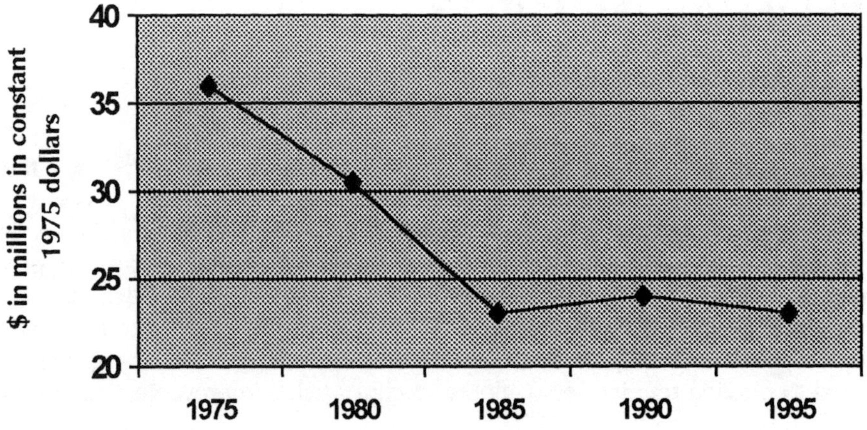

Source: Centers for Disease Control, 1996.

Centers for Disease Control and Prevention

The Division of STD Prevention at the Centers for Disease Control and Prevention provides national leadership through research, policy development, and support of effective services to prevent STDs, including HIV. The division's goals are to reduce the health complications caused by STDs, including enhanced HIV transmission, infertility, adverse outcomes of pregnancy, and reproductive tract cancer.

The majority of the CDC's STD prevention funds are allocated to state and local health departments for prevention and control efforts at the state and local levels. (Appendix A contains details about CDC's national efforts in STD prevention and control.)

The Division of STD Prevention also is responsible for achieving the objectives assigned to it by the Public Health Service by the year 2000 as they relate to STD prevention and control. The executive branch mandated a national collaboration effort led by the Public Health Service—Healthy People 2000—where health professionals, citizens, private organizations and public agencies are working to improve the health of Americans by the year 2000. STD was determined to be one of the 22 priority health areas that needs improvement in the United States.

Table 10. Federal STD Appropriation History, 1970 –1998

Year	Grant	Direct Operations	Total
1970	$6,333,094	$5,314,000	$11,647,094
1971	6,300,000	5,834,000	12,134,000
1972	22,300,000	5,930,000	28,230,000
1973	24,800,000	6,540,000	31,340,000
1974	24,800,000	7,513,000	32,313,000
1975	28,000,000	8,230,000	36,230,000
1976	19,840,000	8,524,000	28,364,000
1977	25,000,000	9,875,000	34,875,000
1978	32,000,000	9,875,000	41,875,000
1979	32,000,000	7,056,000	39,056,000
1980	35,034,000	7,801,000	47,801,000
1981	39,100,000	8,002,000	47,102,000
1982	35,419,000	6,981,000	42,400,000
1983	40,000,000	7,692,000	47,692,000
1984	45,510,000	8,968,000	54,478,000
1985	45,510,000	9,185,000	54,695,000
1986	44,511,000	9,354,000	53,865,000
1987	50,000,000	9,943,000	59,943,000
1988	54,572,000	10,589,000	65,161,000
1989	68,172,000	10,528,000	78,700,000
1990	70,666,000	10,640,000	81,306,000
1991	73,638,000	11,330,000	84,968,000
1992	77,525,000	11,296,000	88,821,000
1993	78,042,000	11,510,000	89,552,000
1994	86,461,000	13,310,000	99,771,000
1995	91,838,000	13,326,000	105,164,000
1996	91,938,100	13,303,400	105,241,500
1997	90,364,252	15,838,748	106,203,000
1998	97,412,252	16,258,748	113,671,000

Source: Centers for Disease Control and Prevention, Division of STD Prevention. 1998.

Infertility Appropriations*

1994	$8,300,000
1995	$12,200,000
1996	$12,783,700
1997	$13,076,919
1998	$17,634,919

*Included in grants figure above.
Source: Centers for Disease Control and Prevention, Division of STD Prevention, 1998.

National Institutes of Health

The National Institutes of Health (NIH) is one of the world's foremost biomedical research centers and the federal focal point for biomedical research in the United States. It is one of the eight health agencies of the federal Public Health Service within the U.S. Department of Health and Human Services. The goal of NIH is to acquire new knowledge to help prevent, detect, diagnose, and treat disease and disability, from the rarest genetic disorder to the common cold.

The NIH budget which was about $300 in 1887, today totals more than $13.6 billion. Within the National Institute of Allergy and Infectious Diseases (NIAID) at NIH is the Division of Microbiology and Infectious Disease, Sexually Transmitted Disease Branch. Its mission is to foster, develop and administer a research program that will contribute to the reproductive health of people and specifically lead to prevention and control of STDs. Like the CDC, the division's goals are to prevent infertility, adverse pregnancy outcomes, reproductive tract tumors, other chronic STD consequences and HIV infection. Incorporating biomedical, behavioral, clinical and epidemiological research efforts is the central theme of NIAID programs.

6. STD PREVENTION PROGRAMS

Prevention programs address sexually transmitted diseases at all levels—local, state and national—and each program plays a different and critical role in STD prevention. Behavioral researchers observe that people do not, in general, respond to the same message. It is, therefore, important to provide programs that are appropriate to various ages, cultures, and education levels.

The debate continues about what prevention messages should be taught. Should specific values and behaviors be taught? Should courses focus solely on abstinence, or should they also include how to use a condom?

Abstinence-Based Programs

Beginning in fiscal year 1998, Congress appropriated $50 million annually for the next five years. The money goes to states to promote the abstinence until marriage message through school and community prevention programs. Although some criticize the program, a significant amount of data and medical opinion supports abstinence programs.[42] Content of the programs varies, but the message remains the same, emphasizing sexual abstinence outside a mutually monogamous, lifelong relationship.

School Programs to Reduce Sexual Risk Behaviors

A review of school-affiliated programs designed to reduce sexual risk behavior found, in some cases, that they delayed the initiation of intercourse, reduced the frequency of intercourse, reduced the number of sexual partners, or increased the use of condoms or other contraceptives. Effective programs give a clear and narrow message, "Delay having sex, but if you do have sex, always use a condom."[43] According to the Sexuality Information and Education Council of the United States (SIECUS), at least 36 states have laws mandating HIV education in schools. Twenty-two states have laws requiring schools to discuss disease prevention methods.

Innovations in STD Education: Model Program Search

This national search for community-based programs, designed to reduce the incidence of STDs, was sponsored in 1997 by 3M Pharmaceuticals. A panel of national STD education, prevention, treatment and research experts reviewed 47 programs and identified the winners. Criteria for the winning programs included program excellence, degree of innovation and replicability.

- ***Entre Nosotros***, an STD Accelerated Prevention Campaign Project, is sponsored by the Planned Parenthood Association of Hidalgo County in McAllen, Texas. The program focuses on Mexican American women and men of reproductive age with an additional focus on teens. Twenty-eight men, women and teens from the rural area carry out a door-to-door peer education program designed to reduce STDs among Hidalgo County residents by 20 percent by 1998. Results since 1996 show that the peer educators traveled 28,589 miles to reach 9,635 adults and 4,243 teens with their reproductive health education, family planning counseling, and STD and HIV prevention messages. Referrals and follow-ups were completed for 159 high-risk people and additional 67 at-risk pregnant women were identified and tested for syphilis during each trimester of their pregnancies.

- **The Prevention Connection**, sponsored by the Los Angeles County Department of Health Services STD Program, is a partnership between the STD program and pharmacists, beauticians and barbers in Los Angeles County areas that have high STD rates. The program targets high-risk Los Angeles County residents who have little or no contact with the health care system, but who frequent pharmacies and salons or barbershops. Participating establishments provide answers to their client's questions about STDs. In addition, clients have access to free condoms. Participating businesses are STD prevention advocates within the community who provide free information packets and clinic referrals. Project results show an increase in reported condom use, an increase in patronage for businesses that are part of the project, and an increase in discussions with the pharmacists, beauticians and barbers about HIV/AIDS and STDs.

- **Youth in Action**, a program in Denver, Colorado, is sponsored by Denver Public Health. The program targets high-risk youth of color in central Denver, specifically young women, due to the higher risk of complications associated with STDs and women. The screening project, part of Youth in Action, is called Peers for Education and Enhanced Screening Project (PEES). The program recruits and trains peer volunteers to target youth who may need a referral to outreach workers for urine chlamydia screening. Outreach workers collect demographic information, the young person's history of STDs, current sexual risk behavior, and factors associated with their barriers to care. Partners of those who test positive are contacted, encouraged to seek further screening and treatment, and referred to a local clinic. More than 800 screening tests have been performed since the program's inception in the spring of 1994. Approximately 20 percent of those tested were young women. Of the 6.6 percent of people who have tested positive, the majority had no symptoms of infection.

Programs that received honorable mention in the search were: "Condom Promotion Interventions for STD Clinic Patients," sponsored by the Boston University School of Public Health; "STD Case Management Project," sponsored by the Cook County (Ill.) Department of Public Health; "Brown Bag Special Condom Availability," under the auspices of Planned Parenthood of Austin, Texas; Planned Parenthood of Greater Cleveland's "H.I.P. Program;" "Live Wire Youth Conference," a program through Planned Parenthood of El Paso, Texas; "Deaf Community HIV/AIDS + STD Network," sponsored by St. Paul, Minnesota's Deafness Education Advocacy Foundation; "BASE (Be Active in Self Education) Grants," and the HIV/AIDS Technical Assistance Program in Brooklyn, New York.

Innovations in Syphilis Prevention Project

The "Innovations in Syphilis Prevention Project" in Houston, Texas, is a community-based STD program that specifically targets syphilis. The program was designed as a partnership between the School of Public Health at the University of Texas at Houston, the City of Houston Department of Health and Human Services, and Over the Hill Inc.—a nonprofit community-based organization. The targeted communities for the project are those with high incidence of syphilis and inner-city neighborhoods with high rates of poverty, unemployment and large minority populations. The purpose of the project is to increase knowledge about syphilis, increase screening rates, and decrease rates of syphilis cases through prevention and early treatment. The primary intervention methods are fliers, billboard advertisements, and a video with stories focusing on role models. Peer outreach workers, a mobile van, neighborhood businesses, and private physicians distribute the fliers along with a condom. No information is yet available about the program's effectiveness.

School-Based Chlamydia Control Program

A Louisiana program conducted by researchers from Louisiana State University, Tulane University, and the Louisiana Department of Public Health investigated the feasibility of a school-based chlamydia control program. Beginning in 1995, all of the students at three inner-city New Orleans junior/senior high schools, regardless of symptoms or sexual history, were given the opportunity to be tested for chlamydia following individual counseling regarding the test. Students had to obtain parental consent either for school clinic services or for the chlamydia test in order to participate in the urine-based testing. The only way parents could obtain the test results was from their child. Testing took place during five three-week testing periods.

The new availability of urine tests provides an opportunity to screen large numbers of people (in this case, high school students) for chlamydia in a noninvasive manner. The urine tests for chlamydia (polymerase chain reaction [PCR] and ligase chain reaction [LCR]) are sensitive and easy to use.

Researchers obtained parental consent from 86.9 percent of the parents of students in grades 7 through 12 and tested 59 percent of the students enrolled in the three schools. Results concluded that the girls tested positive for chlamydia more than twice as often as the boys, but girls were less likely to be tested than boys. Rates generally increased with age. Students who were infected were counseled and offered oral treatment with azithromycin and referred or offered additional testing for other STDs. They also were asked to let their sexual partners know that they should be treated. The positivity rates for both boys and girls consistently decreased for each of the past three years.

The investigators in this study concluded that school-based testing is feasible and has a high success rate. The laboratory cost for testing was relatively inexpensive—$17.76 per test. The cost of treatment per infected student was a little more than $200.[44] No information is yet available regarding the effectiveness of the program, but there has been a consecutive decrease in the positivity rate annually since 1995.

California Partnership for Adolescent Chlamydia Prevention

The California Department of Health Services recently initiated the California Partnership for Adolescent Chlamydia Prevention. The statewide partnership brings together government agencies, managed care organizations, academic health centers and professional associations to address policy issues relating to adolescents and STDs. Other components of the initiative include development of screening, counseling and education interventions, media campaigns aimed at adolescents, school-based programs and health care provider training programs.[45]

National Programs

In 1993, Congress appropriated funds to begin a national STD-related infertility prevention program. Through a cooperative effort between the CDC and the Office of Population Affairs, the program involves strong collaboration among family planning, STD and primary health care programs, and public health laboratories.[46]

In addition to the Public Health Service (PHS) Region X demonstration project discussed below, other PHS regions have successfully implemented infertility prevention programs. These regions have noted decreases in the rates of chlamydia among women although their programs have not been in existence as long as the Region X program. Federal Region III (Delaware, the District of Columbia, Maryland, Pennsylvania, Virginia and West Virginia) noted a 31 percent decline in infection in females under age 20 during the first two and one-half years of initial large-scale screening, which began in 1994. Region VIII (Colorado, Montana, North Dakota, South Dakota, Utah and Wyoming) noted a 16 percent decline in infection for females under age 20 during the first two and one half years of initial screening. The national program continues as a demonstration project due to resource and budget constraints.[47]

Chlamydia and its consequences cost the United States more than $2 billion per year. The CDC estimates that screening and treatment programs can be conducted at an annual cost of $175 million.[48]

Region X Chlamydia Project—A Partnership for Prevention of Infertility

The Public Health Region X (Alaska, Idaho, Oregon, and Washington) Chlamydia Project is a national model for reaching women who are at risk of acquiring chlamydia infection. The program began in 1988 with 150 family planning clinics and expanded in 1993 to STD clinics and other health agencies. The program now operates in about 500 community-based health agencies that provide services to adult and adolescent females throughout the Pacific Northwest.

Significant progress has been made where chlamydia screening programs have been fully implemented. The Region X Chlamydia Project resulted in a 62 percent decline in infection among women tested between 1988 and 1997 (see table 11).

Since 1988, more than 700,000 women have been tested for chlamydia through this program. In family planning clinics, from 1988 to 1997, a 62 percent reduction in disease was seen in all the Region X states throughout all age groups. During the past 10 years, 100,000 women and their partners were treated. More than $4 million was saved in 1997 by preventing costly medical complications. At least 48,000 teenage women have been successfully treated for chlamydial infections.

Collaboration is a key component of the program. Partnerships among state and local agencies throughout Region X save at least $1 million annually. One dollar spent on screening and treatment saves $12 in costs for treatment of future complications.[49]

**Table 11. Region X Chlamydia Project Results
1988 – 1997, by Region/State**

Chlamydia Positivity – Female Clients, by Region/State					
Family Planning Clinics Percent of Chlamydia Positive			STD Clinics Percent of Chlamydia Positive		
1988	1997	Percent Decline	1993	1997	Percent Decline
Region X 9.3%	3.5%	62%	7.1%	5.3%	25%
STATE					
Alaska 12.2	3.0	75	9	6.5	18
Idaho 10.5	3.5	67	7.8	7.2	8
Oregon 8.9	2.9	67	6.9	5.5	20
Washington 9.3	3.8	59	7.1	4.8	32

Chlamydia Positivity – Female Clients, by Age or Group					
Family Planning Clinics Percent of Chlamydia Positive			STD Clinics Percent of Chlamydia Positive		
1988	1997	Percent Decline	1993	1997	Percent Decline
AGE GROUP					
Teens 12.2	4.6	62	13.6	8.8	35
20-24 8.5	3.0	65	6.8	5.8	15
25+ 4.1	2.0	51	2.5	2.1	16

Source: Region X Infertility Prevention Project, 1997.

Georgia Chlamydia Screening

House Bill 1565 was introduced during the 1998 legislative session in the Georgia House of Representatives. Signed by Governor Zell Miller, Chapter 17 of Title 31 of the Official Code of Georgia Annotated requires coverage of optional annual chlamydia screening tests for females who are covered by individual or group accident and sickness insurance policies or managed care plans. The law, which became effective on July 1, 1998, is the first of its kind. It could serve as a model for state efforts to reduce and prevent chlamydial infection and mitigate the long-term costs and consequences associated with untreated infection.

7. RECOMMENDATIONS FOR STD PREVENTION AND TREATMENT

According to the Centers for Disease Control and Prevention, STD prevention and treatment programs are based on five primary activities:

- Education of those at risk about how to reduce the risk of STDs;

- Detection of people who are infected but have no symptoms, and of people who are infected and have symptoms but who are not likely to seek diagnostic and treatment services;

- Effective diagnosis and treatment of infected people;

- Evaluation, treatment and counseling of sex partners of people who are infected with an STD;

- Preexposure vaccination of people who are at risk for vaccine-preventable STDs like Hepatitis A and B.[50] (Hepatitis A is more commonly transmitted through foodborne viruses, but can be transmitted sexually.)

Prevention Programs

The Institute of Medicine (IOM), the health policy arm of the National Academy of Sciences, convened a 16-member committee of health experts to study the issue of STDs and make recommendations for solutions to the problem. Results of the 18-month study were published in *The Hidden Epidemic: Confronting Sexually Transmitted Diseases* in 1997. Recognizing the absence of a systematic approach to STD prevention in the United States, the committee recommended that "an effective national system for STD prevention be established in the United States."[51] The committee also recommended four strategies to establish an effective national system for preventing STDs. The strategies stress open communication; strong leadership; targeting adolescents and underserved populations, such as substance users, people in detention facilities, prostitutes, the homeless and migrant workers; and access to essential clinical services.

The four recommendations provide a glimpse of the work that the committee believes needs to be done to develop a national effective system for preventing STDs.

1. *Overcome barriers to healthy sexual behaviors.*

   According to the IOM report, an array of biological, social and structural factors impede STD prevention efforts. The committee reports that, by more openly confronting issues of sexuality and STDs, many of these obstacles to prevention could be overcome. Open communication at all relationship levels—parent and child, sex partners, media, at school, in the community—is an important aspect of learning about and understanding healthy sexual behavior. This means talking about sex in a positive way that fosters healthy sexuality and educates people about both the gains and the losses involved in any sexual relationship from the physical, emotional, spiritual, intellectual and financial aspects.

2. *Develop strong leadership, strengthen investment and improve information systems for STD prevention.*

To establish a national STD prevention system, leadership and support for STD prevention must be improved at all levels of the private and public sectors, especially among elected officials. Public agencies have neither the resources nor the capabilities to implement a national system, so the private sector should be involved to help make up the difference.

The committee recommends that federal, state and local elected officials provide additional funding for STD prevention.

3. *Design and implement essential STD-related services in innovative ways for adolescents and underserved populations.*

These populations were targeted because they are at highest risk and are the most in need of STD-related services. Innovative ways to reach youth and disenfranchised populations (e.g. substance users, people in detention facilities, sex workers, the homeless, and migrant workers) need to be created to focus on their particular needs.

4. *Ensure access to and quality of essential clinical services for STDs.*

Several suggestions are provided to improve access and quality of care as they relate to STD services. Those include ensuring access to services in the community, improving dedicated public STD clinics, involving health plans and purchasers of health care, improving training and education of health care professionals, and improving clinical management of STDs.

Treatment Programs

In addition, the IOM committee cited a lack of appropriate screening and treatment as a factor that contributes to the STD epidemic in the United States. The panel concluded that patients who are diagnosed often receive inadequate treatment or treatment that is inconsistent with recommended practice. The CDC's *1998 Guidelines for Treatment of Sexually Transmitted Disease* updates the 1993 CDC recommendations for STD screening, diagnosis and treatment. The recommendations were developed by CDC staff in consultation with national STD experts from public health, academia, and medical research and managed care organizations.

Some advances made since publication of CDC's guidelines include the highly effective single-dose oral therapies that have been developed for almost all common curable STDs; improved treatments for herpes and human papillomavirus (HPV); urine tests; Hepatitis A and B vaccinations for all sexually active youth; and improved treatment for STDs in pregnancy.[50]

8. SUMMARY OF STATE LAWS

Policymakers will find it fascinating to consider the kinds of STD laws that have endured throughout our nation's history that address prevention, testing and treatment for STDs. Of particular interest to lawmakers today will be the sections on informed consent, testing for pregnant women and prisoners, reporting and notification, and confidentiality.

The summary of STD statutes covers issues relating to administration; confidentiality; consent for release of records; counseling; court proceedings and penalties; STD definitions; education; prevention; funding; Hepatitis B; investigation; notification; quarantining; compulsory testing and treatment; reporting for gonorrhea; syphilis and other STDs; sexual assault and sexual offenders; testing for gonorrhea, chlamydia and other STDs; testing for pregnant women and newborns; prisoner testing; treatment; and miscellaneous issues.

The summaries of STD statutes are provided as information to policymakers and others about laws that exist in the 50 states, commonwealths and territories through 1997. The statutes initially were identified by a WESTLAW database search. Researchers also combed the indices of the statutes to identify laws that specifically target sexually transmitted disease or venereal disease. The summary includes HIV/AIDS laws only when they include mention of sexually transmitted diseases. In addition to state laws, many STD clinical, operational and other policies exist in departmental regulations.

A recent publication, *Improving State Law to Prevent and Treat Infectious Disease,*[52] contends that there is a need for reform of public health laws, including many STD laws. The report describes how some laws are outdated and have not kept up with scientific technology, including current treatment. It asserts that many laws have not been updated with regard to the current interpretation of constitutional limits on states' authority to restrict individual liberties. The report recommends that STD laws avoid disease-specific provisions so they are not so limiting, and take into account emerging diseases.

The report also advises stronger protection for individual privacy.[53] Yet, a more recent argument contends that many laws afford too much protection for the STD-infected person and not enough for the unknowingly exposed partner. According to the report:

> Nevertheless, it is important to be candid about the limits of the legislative approach when considering reform of STD laws. Many of the problems in public health can be remedied through better leadership and training, improved infrastructure for surveillance and epidemiological investigations, and innovative prevention strategies. The law is only one factor that guides public health officials. Communicable disease law still must be applied in the real world. In making policy decisions, public health authorities will have to consider prevailing social values and respect multiple constituencies, including scientists, politicians and community activists.[54]

Administrative Requirements

CA   **Cal. Health & Safety Code § 120530 (West 1996)** allows the department to help in treating cases of venereal disease in cities or counties that do not have adequate treatment facilities.

CA   **Cal. Health & Safety Code § 120535 (West 1996)** requires a public hospital to admit acute venereal disease cases that are found to be a menace to public health.

CO   **Colo. Rev. Stat. § 25-4-406 (1997)** requires all department rules and regulations regarding venereal diseases to have the effect of law.

FL   **Fla. Stat. Ann. § 384.22 (West 1993)** describes the intent of the Legislature to provide a program that meets the emerging needs, and deals efficiently and effectively to reduce STDs.

FL   **Fla. Stat. Ann. § 384.281 (West 1993 & Supplemental 1998)** provides the department with guidelines for prehearing detention for an STD-infected person who is considered a threat to public health. Outlines procedures for confining an infected person. Requires an infected person to have a bail hearing within 24 hours.

IL   **Ill. Ann. Stat. ch. 410 § 325/10 (Smith-Hurd 1997)** requires the department to adopt the rules necessary to perform the duties of the department. Requires rules of the department to include criteria, standards and procedures for the identification, investigation, examination and treatment of STDs.

LA   **La. Rev. Stat. Ann § 1300.71 (West Supplemental 1998)** requires the department to prepare an annual health report card indicating the overall state of health in Louisiana. Requires the report card to include state information about teenage pregnancy, birth rates, rates of low birth-weight babies, suicide rates, drug addiction, STDs and other health findings.

LA   **La. Rev. Stat. Ann § 2198.2 (West Supplemental 1998)** requires the rural health care authority to establish six commissions to research, develop and improve the health services for adolescents and special population groups, and reduce STDs and teenage pregnancies.

MA   **Mass. Gen. Laws Ann. ch. 17, § 4 (West 1994)** requires there be, within the department, the establishment of a Division of Communicable and Venereal Disease, which is responsible for the prevention and control of communicable and venereal diseases and the provision of diagnostic and treatment care of those having or suspected of having a venereal disease.

MT   **Mont. Code Ann. § 50-18-103 (1997)** requires the department to cooperate with federal agencies regarding the prevention, control and treatment of STDs. Allows the department to expend federal funds made available to the state for the prevention, control and treatment of STDs.

MT   **Mont. Code Ann. § 50-18-105 (1997)** requires that rules adopted by the department concerning the prevention and control of STDs are binding on all persons and have the effect of law.

MT   **Mont. Code Ann. § 50-18-107 (1997)** outlines powers and duties of health officers. Authorizes health officers to examine, isolate, or investigate a person suspected of being infected with an STD. Allows only a local or state health officer to terminate a quarantine.

OK   **Okla. Stat. Ann. tit. 63, § 1-236 (1997)** defines terms used in administering the state plan. Declares that the purpose of the plan is to provide a comprehensive, coordinated, multidisciplinary and interagency effort to reduce the rate of adolescent pregnancy and STDs in the state.

OK   **Okla. Stat. Ann. tit. 63, § 1-237 (1997)** creates the Joint Legislative Committee for Review of Coordination of Efforts for Prevention of Adolescent Pregnancy and STDs and the Interagency Coordinating Council for Coordination of Efforts for Prevention of Adolescent Pregnancy. Outlines appointment requirements for the committees, duties and objectives. Requires the joint committee to meet with state officials and employees responsible for providing services relating to the prevention of adolescent pregnancy and STDs on a regular basis, evaluate successful programs throughout the nation, recommend changes in proposed interagency agreements and the state plan, review interagency agreements and the state plan, hold hearings regarding STDs and teen pregnancy, monitor and implement the state plan, and recommend legislation to correct any upcoming problems in implementing the plan.

OK   **Okla. Stat. Ann. tit. 63, § 1-238 (1997)** creates coordination of efforts for the prevention of adolescent pregnancy and STDs. Requires the plan be a comprehensive, coordinated, multidisciplinary and interagency effort to reduce the rate of adolescent pregnancy and STDs in the state. Requires components of the plan to include a public awareness campaign, identification of prevention strategies and resources, coordination and collaboration among related efforts and programs, empowerment of local community prevention efforts, and evaluation of prevention strategies and programs. Requires the public awareness campaign to promote abstinence from premarital sex and requires that the campaign cannot directly or indirectly condone premarital or promiscuous sexual activity.

PR   **P.R. Laws Ann. tit. 24, § 579 (1993)** allows the department to establish STD clinics.

PR   **P.R. Laws Ann. tit. 24, § 582 (1993)** authorizes the secretary of health to promulgate any rules or regulations that assist in supporting STD prevention and treatment of efforts.

SC   **S.C. Code Ann. § 44-29-130 (Law. Co-op 1997)** authorizes the department to adopt rules and regulations pertaining to STDs.

VT   **Vt. Stat. Ann. tit. 18, § 1100 (1982)** requires the board to make and enforce any rule or regulation for quarantining and treating any reported venereal disease cases for the protection of the public.

WA   **Wash. Rev. Code Ann. § 70.24.005 (1996)** transfers the duties of control and treatment of STDs and public health safety to the department from other state departments.

WA   **Wash. Rev. Code Ann. § 70.24.015 (1996)** declares that STDs constitute an increasingly serious and sometimes fatal threat to the state's public welfare. Requires all programs designed to deal with STDs meet patient's privacy, confidentiality and dignity. Requires the state to make programs that meet emerging needs and operate efficiently and effectively while reducing the incidence of STDs. Mandates all information be confidential.

WA   **Wash. Rev. Code Ann. § 70.24.130 (1996)** authorizes the board to adopt rules to implement and enforce regulating STDs. Requires the rules to protect the confidentiality of persons investigated and records.

WA   **Wash. Rev. Code Ann. § 70. 24.150 (1996)** provides immunity from civil action for state and local boards of health members, public health officers, and employees of the department for damages arising from the performance of their duties in regulating STDs, unless in gross negligence.

WI   **Wis. Stat. Ann. § 252.10 (West Supplemental 1997)** requires a physician to notify the department when an STD-infected person refuses or stops treatment. Authorizes the department to take the necessary steps to have the person committed for treatment or observation. Allows the court to commit to treatment persons who refuse. Outlines court procedures.

WI   **Wis. Stat. Ann. § 252.10 (West Supplemental 1997)** requires programs in counties that have an incidence of gonorrhea, chlamydia or syphilis that exceeds the statewide average, to diagnose and treat STDs at no cost to the patient. Requires the county board of supervisors to be responsible for ensuring that the program exists, but boards are required to establish their own programs only if no other public or private program is operating. Requires the department to compile statistics indicating the incidence of gonorrhea, chlamydia and syphilis for each county in the state.

WY   **Wyo. Stat. § 35-4-130 (1997)** requires the department to develop a list of reportable STDs. Requires the list be available to all physicians, health officers, hospitals and other health care providers and facilities within the state.

Confidentiality

AL   **Ala. Code § 22-11A-14 (1997)** outlines reporting procedures for STDs. Requires a physician who diagnoses or treats STDs to report to the state or county health officer. Requires laboratories to report all positive or reactive STD tests. Requires all reports and documentation be confidential. Makes it a misdemeanor for violating any reporting rules with a penalty ranging from $100 to $500 upon conviction.

AL   **Ala. Code § 22-11A-22 (1997)** maintains that all records are confidential and cannot be used against the patient. Release of records is allowed only with the written consent of the patient. Makes it a Class C misdemeanor for medical records of infected persons to be released without written consent of the patient.

AK   **Alaska Stat. § 18.15.310** requires that all blood drawn for a court-ordered HIV or STD test of a person charged with a sex offense be performed by a physician, physician's assistant or other qualified personnel and tested in a medically approved laboratory. Requires all test results that indicate exposure to or infection by HIV or other STDs be reported to the department. Requires anyone who receives test results, other than the test subjects, maintain confidentiality. Requires the department provide free counseling and free testing to the victim for HIV and other STDs and counseling to the alleged sex offender upon request of the offender. Requires the department to provide referral to appropriate health care facilities and support services at the request of the victim.

AR   **Ark. Stat. Ann. § 20-16-504 (1991)** requires all laboratory reports be confidential and not open for public inspection except by public health personnel.

CA   **Cal. Health & Safety Code § 120705 (West 1996)** maintains confidentiality of reports. Requires all reports be confidential and not accessible to public inspection.

CA   **Cal. Health & Safety Code § 125105 (West 1996)** requires that Hepatitis B test results remain confidential.

CT   **Conn. Gen. Stat. § 19a-216 (1997)** allows any municipal health department, state institution or facility, licensed physician or any public or private hospital or clinic to examine and treat a minor for a venereal disease. Requires the records of the exam and treatment of the minor be confidential and not be divulged by the facility or physician, including prohibiting sending the bill for services to any person other than the minor. Requires the minor be responsible for all costs and expenses for services. Requires reporting any venereal disease treatment of a minor less than 12 years old to the commissioner of children and families.

DE   **Del. Code Ann. tit. 16, § 702 (1996)** outlines the reporting procedures for STDs. Requires any physician who diagnoses or treats STDs to report to the state or county health officer. Requires any lab that conducts STD testing report all positive or reactive tests. Requires all reports and documentation be held confidential. Authorizes the state or county to follow appropriate procedures for infection control.

DE   **Del. Code Ann. tit. 16, § 710 (1996)** outlines the protocol for treatment, consent and liability for payment in the care of minors for STDs. Requires records be confidential.

DE   **Del. Code Ann. tit. 16, § 711 (1996)** maintains confidentiality of records and information. Allows records to be released for statistical purposes when the person's identity is anonymous and with the consent of all persons identified when enforcing the rules of the department concerning the control and treatment of STDs, in case of a medical emergency, and during civil and criminal litigation. Outlines the procedures for releasing confidential information during court proceedings.

DE   **Del. Code Ann. tit. 16, § 712 (1996)** prohibits public health officials from disclosing any information about the records of a person infected or being treated for STDs or HIV without the consent of that person.

DC   **D. C. Stat. Code Ann. § 30-120 (1997)** requires information about a syphilis laboratory blood test required for a marriage license be confidential by any person, agency or committee who obtains, transmits or receives any information.

FL   **Fla. Stat. Ann. § 384.22 (West 1993)** describes the intent of the Legislature to provide a program that meets the emerging needs, and deals efficiently and effectively at reducing STDs, and provides patients with the knowledge that their information will remain confidential.

FL   **Fla. Stat. Ann. § 384.26 (West 1993 and Supplemental 1998)** authorizes the department to investigate any person infected or suspected of being infected with an STD. Requires all information collected during the investigation be confidential.

FL   **Fla. Stat. Ann. § 384.282 (West 1993 and Supplemental 1998)** requires all court decisions, orders, petitions and other formal documents be protected and confidential. Requires the name of an infected person be protected in court by providing a fake name. Requires any court proceeding where the true name was used be sealed.

FL   **Fla. Stat. Ann. § 384.287 (West 1998)** allows for an officer, firefighter or paramedic who may have been exposed to an STD in the line of duty to request testing of the person they were exposed to as well as be tested themselves. Allows for a court order if the suspected person does not volunteer for testing. States that results are exempt from confidentiality.

FL   **Fla. Stat. Ann. § 384.29 (West 1998)** maintains confidentiality of records and information held by the department or authorized representatives. Authorizes information to be released only when the infected person gives consent and data are used for statistical information and the person is not identified; for medical personnel, state agencies or courts to enforce the law; and for a medical emergency. Exempts medical personnel from any liability.

FL   **Fla. Stat. Ann. § 384.30 (West 1998)** outlines the protocol for the treatment and consent in the care of minors for STDs. Requires that consultation, examination and treatment of a minor for an STD remain confidential.

FL   **Fla. Stat. Ann. § 384.33 (West 1993)** allows the department to adopt rules regarding the investigation, treatment and confidentiality of STDs.

FL   **Fla. Stat. Ann. § 384.34 (West 1993 and Supplemental 1998)** makes it a misdemeanor of the first degree when any person infected with an STD or HIV engages in sexual acts with a nonconsenting person or a person who is not informed of the infection. Makes it a misdemeanor of the first degree to break confidentiality during an STD investigation. Makes it a misdemeanor of the second degree for any person found of guilty of giving false information about the existence of an STD. Requires that a person who violates the rules of the department regarding STDs be fined no more than $500 for each violation.

FL   **Fla. Stat. Ann. § 385.25 (West 1998)** requires any person who diagnoses a person with an STD and any laboratory that conducts a positive STD test result to report the diagnosis to the department within two weeks. Requires the department to adopt rules specifying the information required and a minimum time period for reporting STDs. Requires the department to consider the need for information, privacy and confidentiality of the patient, and the practical ability of authorized personnel and labs to report in a reasonable fashion.

GA   **Ga. Code Ann. § 42-1-7 (1997)** requires any state or county correctional institution, municipal or county detention facility to notify the law enforcement agency of the transporting of an inmate or patient infected with any venereal disease, HIV or other infectious, communicable disease. Requires information released for the transporting be kept confidential and only be released or obtained by the institution, facilities or agencies that are involved with the transporting of the infected patient or inmate. Makes it a misdemeanor for any person to make any unauthorized disclosure of the transporting information.

HI   **Hawaii Rev. Stat. § 325-54 (1993)** maintains confidentiality of reports and outlines the penalties for violating confidentiality. Requires any person breaking confidentiality be fined $500 or imprisoned for no more than 90 days or both.

ID   **Idaho Code § 39-604 (Supplemental 1997)** requires testing and treating any person for a venereal disease and HIV imprisoned in any state correctional facility. Requires testing and treating any person for a venereal disease confined in any county or city jail when public health officials think there was exposure to an infection. Requires testing any person, including a juvenile, for HIV and Hepatitis B when charged with a sex offense or prostitution. Requires the court to release the test results to the victim or to the parent or guardian when the victim is a minor. Requires a prisoner to be entitled to HIV counseling when tested HIV positive and to receive referrals to appropriate health care and support services. Requires the victim to receive counseling and referral services at the time of the test results.

ID   **Idaho Code § 39-606 (1993)** requires all reports regarding venereal disease be confidential. Makes it a misdemeanor for any person who willfully or maliciously discloses the contents of any confidential public health record except under written authorization by the infected person who is on the record.

ID   **Idaho Code § 39-1004 (1993)** provides guidelines in reporting laboratory tests. Requires laboratories to furnish a detailed report and result of the serological syphilis test. Requires a laboratory not operated by the department to file a report with the department. Maintains that reports are kept confidential and not open for public inspection.

IL   **Ill. Ann. Stat. ch. 410 § 325/2 (Smith-Hurd 1997)** states the General Assembly's findings and intent that all programs designed to deal with STDs will provide patients with privacy, confidentiality and dignity. The state's intent is to provide a program that is sufficiently flexible to meet emerging needs, deals efficiently and effectively with reducing the incidence of STDs, and provides patients with a secure knowledge that the information they provide will remain private and confidential.

IL   **Ill. Ann. Stat. ch. 410 § 325/5 (Smith-Hurd 1997)** requires the department to adopt rules regarding the authorization of interviews for investigating persons infected or believed to be infected with an STD, and to order a person to submit to an examination and treatment. Requires all information gathered during an investigation be confidential. Makes it a Class A misdemeanor for any person who knowingly discloses any information of any person infected with an STD.

IL   **Ill. Ann. Stat. ch. 410 § 325/8 (Smith-Hurd 1997)** requires all reports and documentation of STDs to be confidential. Lists exemptions. Allows information to be used only when consent is given by the individual. Upon receiving a report, the state or county will follow the appropriate procedure for infection control.

IL   **Ill. Ann. Stat. ch. 745, 40/3 (Smith-Hurd 1993)** requires all information about a reported STD case remain confidential and not be publicly disclosed. Requires information about a minor under 11 years of age with a venereal disease be reported in accordance with the Abused and Neglected Child Reporting Act of 1975.

IA   **Iowa Code § 140.4 (1997)** requires reporting immediately after the first examination or treatment of any person infected with any venereal disease. Requires that report to include the name, age, sex, marital status, occupation of patient, name of the disease, probable source of infection and duration of the disease. Requires that reports be confidential. Requires immunity from any civil or criminal liability for any person making a report.

KS   **Kan. Stat. Ann § 65-153f (Supplemental 1997)** requires a physician or a person attending a pregnant woman, with the consent of the woman, to take a blood sample for a serological test for syphilis and Hepatitis B within 14 days after the diagnosis of pregnancy. Requires an approved laboratory report all positive or reactive tests. Requires all laboratory reports, files and records to be confidential and only be opened by authorized health officers or by written consent of the woman.

KY   **Ky. Rev. Stat. § 214.420 (1995)** declares confidentiality is essential for the proper control and prevention of STDs. Requires all information and reports regarding a person infected with or suspected of being infected with an STD be confidential. Specifies only authorized health department personnel who are assigned to STD control activities have access to records and reports. Allows for medical information to be released to the physician of a person suspected of being infected, for statistical purposes where the individual is not identified, with written consent from the person for the information to be released, and in case of a medical emergency.

MA   **Mass. Gen. Laws Ann. ch. 111, § 119 (West 1996)** requires hospitals and laboratories with morbidity reports and records pertaining to a venereal disease not be public record and the contents not to be divulged by any person having access, except under court order or to an authorized person. Makes it a violation for the first offense and punishable by a fine of no more than $50, and each subsequent offense by a fine of no more than $100.

MI   **Mich. Stat. Ann. § 14.15 (5111) (Law. Co-op 1995)** authorizes the department to establish reporting requirements for serious communicable diseases. Allows the department to require a licensed health professional or health facility to report a serious communicable disease or infection within 24 hours of diagnosis. Requires local health departments to furnish care for tuberculosis and venereal diseases. Requires the department to provide rules for the confidentiality of reports, records and data pertaining to the testing, care, treatment, reporting and research associated with tuberculosis, Hepatitis B and other venereal diseases.

MI   **Mich. Stat. Ann. § 14.15 (5121) (Law. Co-op 1995)** makes it a misdemeanor for a county clerk to issue a marriage license to an individual who fails to present a certificate stating the applicant has received counseling about venereal diseases and HIV and has been offered venereal disease and HIV testing. Makes it a misdemeanor for any person who discloses the marriage license applicant has taken a venereal disease or HIV test and discloses the results of the tests except when required by law. Makes it a misdemeanor for a physician who knowingly and willfully makes a false statement in a certificate required for a marriage license.

MI   **Mich. Stat. Ann. § 14.15 (5131) (Law. Co-op 1995)** requires all reports, records and data pertaining to the testing, treatment, reporting and research of venereal diseases, HIV/AIDS and other serious communicable diseases be confidential. Makes it a misdemeanor for any person who violates confidentiality and is punishable by a imprisonment of no more than one year, or a fine of not more than $5,000, or both.

MS   **Miss. Code Ann. § 41-23-30 (1993)** requires the county health departments to provide free testing and treatment for STDs. Requires all testing and treatment be held confidential. Requires using available media to advertise the confidentiality of the test and treatment.

MO   **Mo. Ann. Stat. § 210.040 (Vernon 1996)** requires reporting any positive syphilis or Hepatitis B tests to the department. Requires the report to be held confidential.

MT   **Mont. Code Ann. § 50-19-108 (1997)** requires all laboratory reports be confidential and not open to inspection by any person other than the patient, those designated by the patient to receive the information, or state and local health officers. Any person who divulges this information or inspects any reports without authority to any unauthorized person is guilty of a misdemeanor and may be fined no more than $100.

MT   **Mont. Code Ann. § 50-18-109 (1997)** outlines the release of information when permitted. Allows information concerning a person infected or suspected to be infected with an STD to be released only to authorized personnel of the department, to a physician who has written consent of the person whose record is requested, or to a local health officer engaged in the eradication of STDs. Specifies the importance of protecting and preserving the principle of confidentiality.

NE   **Neb. Rev. Stat. § 71- 502.04 (1996)** outlines reporting procedures. Requires each report supply date, name, result of test performed and, when available, age of the person. Requires name and address of physician requesting test. Requires all laboratory reports be held confidential and not open to public inspection with certain exceptions.

NE   **Neb. Rev. Stat. § 71- 506 (1996)** makes it a Class V misdemeanor for any person who violates any STD rule or regulation of the department. Makes it a Class III misdemeanor for any person who willfully or maliciously breaks confidentiality and discloses the contents of any report, notification or investigation of an STD.

NV   **Nev. Rev. Stat. § 441A.220 (1997)** requires all information regarding the report of an STD case or the investigation of a case by the health authority be confidential and not disclosed to any person, including information used for court proceedings with exceptions. Provides exceptions.

NH   **N.H. Rev. Stat. Ann. § 141-C:10 (1996)** requires any information or report on any examination, quarantine or treatment of a person infected with a venereal disease to be confidential. Allows for information to be disclosed only for health related research or analysis of data with the identity of the individual not disclosed.

NJ   **N.J. Stat. Ann. § 26:4-41 (West 1996)** prohibits any person from disclosing the name, address or identity of a person known or suspected of having a venereal disease except to the person's physician, the health authority or the court. Prohibits any venereal disease documents or reports be open for public inspection.

NM   **N. M. Stat. Ann. § 24-1-9.4 (1997)** prohibits any person who administers a test for STDs to disclose the identity of the person tested or the result of the test that identifies the subject, unless permitted by the person tested.

NM   **N. M. Stat. Ann. § 24-1-9.5 (1997)** prohibits any person who sees the results of an STD test to disclose the test results to another person, except as authorized. Requires that whenever disclosure is made it is accompanied by a statement stating the disclosure policy and the penalty of a petty misdemeanor for disclosing.

NM   **N. M. Stat. Ann. § 24-1-9.7 (1997)** mandates that any person who makes an unauthorized disclosure of confidential information be found guilty of a petty misdemeanor and sentenced to imprisonment in the county jail for a maximum of six months, or payment of a fine of not more than $500, or both.

NY   **N.Y. Public Health Law § 2301 (McKinney 1993)** allows a health officer to apply to court for an order to examine a person who is refusing to be tested for an STD. Requires all papers pertaining to any proceedings be kept confidential except to those authorized to inspect the report.

NY   **N.Y. Public Health Law § 2306 (McKinney 1993)** requires all STD reports and information be confidential. Allows for information to be disclosed by court order in certain criminal proceedings provided that the subject of the information has waived confidentiality. Allows parents or guardians of minors to waive confidentiality.

NY   **N.Y. Public Health Law § 2309 (McKinney 1993)** makes it a misdemeanor for any person who violates the rules and regulations of the department regarding testing, reporting and confidentiality of STDs.

ND   **N.D. Cent. Code § 23-07.7-02 (1997)** outlines testing procedures for court-ordered testing. Requires testing for HIV and STDs. Requires laboratory to send a copy of test results to the physician who supplies results to defendant and victim, and to the department. Makes it a Class C felony for any person who violates confidentiality.

OK   **Okla. Stat. Ann. tit. 43, § 33 (1990)** outlines the procedure for reporting results of a premarital test for syphilis by the doctor and laboratory. Requires the doctor to file results with the state. Requires the results be confidential and not open to public inspection.

OK   **Okla. Stat. Ann. tit. 43, § 37 (1990)** makes it a misdemeanor for any marriage license applicant, physician, governmental or laboratory representative to misrepresent any facts or break confidentiality about any syphilis record or lab report.

OK   **Okla. Stat. Ann. tit. 63, § 1-525 (1997)** requires all information—including the records and test results of an infected person charged with a sex offense—be confidential and only be disclosed by court order. Allows the victim of the crime to request the results of the examination and test results conducted on the offender. Requires the department to provide free testing to the alleged victim for any venereal or communicable disease when the offender tests positive for any tests. Requires that the testing of the victim be accompanied with pretest and post-test counseling. Requires the state board of health to rule and regulate procedural guidelines for testing sex offenders and releasing records containing the sex offender's test results. Requires the guidelines to respect the rights of the person arrested for the alleged sex offense and the victim of the alleged sex offense.

OK   **Okla. Stat. Ann. tit. 63, § 1-532 (1997)** makes all venereal disease information and reports confidential and not accessible to the public.

PA   **Pa. Cons. Stat. Ann. tit. 23, § 1305 (Purdon 1991)** requires a premarital test for syphilis. Requires no marriage license be issued until a statement signed by a licensed physician has been filed. Requires the statement include whether a syphilis test was given and the result from the laboratory. Requires using the physician's statement within 30 days of issuance for the marriage license. Requires a standard serological test for syphilis be a test approved by the department and be made at an approved laboratory. Requires the test be made free of charge when the applicant is unable to pay and when requested by a physician. Allows for an applicant to appeal to the department when having been denied a physician's statement. Outlines filing requirements for marriage licenses and requires all documents be confidential.

PA   **Pa. Cons. Stat. Ann. tit. 35, § 521.15 (Purdon 1993)** prohibits state and local health authorities from disclosing any STD reports. Allows state and local health authorities to use data contained in disease reports for research purposes.

PR   **P.R. Laws Ann. tit. 24, § 572 (1993)** requires the lab to report within five days along with the name of patient, age, sex, address, and name of doctor. Mandates all reports remain confidential.

PR   **P.R. Laws Ann. tit. 24, § 575a (1993)** mandates that all test results remain confidential except in minimal cases where the offender is confirmed HIV positive.

RI   **R.I. Gen. Laws § 23-11-9 (1996)** requires all records be confidential. Requires that any person who divulges the name or gives any information relating to a person suffering from an STD be imprisoned for no more than six months or fined no more than $250.

SC   **S.C. Code Ann. § 44-29-135 (Law. Co-op 1997)** requires information not be released or made public except with the written consent of persons identified. Allows information to be released for statistical purposes where the individual cannot be identified, and for medical information necessary to enforce the control and treatment of STDs and protect the health of the STD-infected person. Requires reporting the name and the medical information of a minor with no further information required to be released by the department.

SD   **S.D. Codified Laws Ann. § 34-23-2 (1994)** requires a physician or other person who diagnoses or treats a person with a venereal disease to report the case to the department. Requires the identity of the infected individual in the report and investigation be kept confidential and not disclosed to any court.

TN   **Tenn. Code Ann. § 68-10-113 (1996)** requires all records of information held by the department relating to known or suspected cases of STDs be confidential. Requires such information not be released or placed in court documents except under certain circumstances. Requires, under the Tennessee Child Abuse Law, reporting any STD case involving a minor less than 13 years old to the appropriate authorities.

TN   **Tenn. Code Ann. § 68-10-114 (1996)** requires than no state or local department officer be asked in civil, criminal or other proceeding about the existence or contents of pertinent records of a person examined or treated for an STD.

TN   **Tenn. Code Ann. § 68-10-116 (1996)** allows an officer to request an arrested person's blood be tested for the presence of Hepatitis B or HIV if the officer is exposed during the arresting, transporting or processing of a person. Requires testing to occur at a licensed health care facility, with the cost to be paid by the division that employs the law enforcement officer. Requires the test be confidential and allows the officer exposed to request the test results.

TX   **Tex. Health & Safety Code Ann. § 81.090 (Vernon 1992)** requires a physician to take a blood sample of a pregnant woman at the first examination and within 24 hours of the delivery and submit the sample to a certified laboratory for a standard serological test for syphilis and a standard serological test for HIV. Outlines other duties required during the first exam, including distributing information about HIV/AIDS and syphilis, verbally notifying the woman that an HIV test will be performed, and advising the woman that the result of the test is not anonymous and explaining the difference between an anonymous and confidential test. Prohibits the physician from conducting the HIV test if the woman objects to the test. Requires the physician to refer the woman to an anonymous testing site or instruct the woman about anonymous testing methods, if she objects to testing.

UT   **Utah Code Ann. § 26-6-20 (1995)** requires a licensed physician or surgeon to take a blood sample of a pregnant woman within 10 days of her first examination and to submit the sample to an approved laboratory for a standard serological test for syphilis. Allows for religious exemption. Requires a copy of the results be given to the physician and a copy submitted to the department. Requires the test results be kept confidential and not open to public inspection.

UT   **Utah Code Ann. § 26-6-20.5 (1995)** requires all reports regarding the investigation, control and reporting of a venereal disease be confidential.

VT   **Vt. Stat. Ann. tit. 18, § 1099 (1982)** requires all information and reports connected with any person suffering from a venereal disease be confidential and not accessible to the public and that names not be disclosed.

VA   **Va. Code § 32.1-36 (1997)** requires a physician who diagnoses a venereal disease in a child 12 years or younger to report the case to the authorities, unless the physician reasonably believes that the infection was acquired congenitally or by means other than sexual abuse. Requires all information reported be confidential.

WA   **Wash. Rev. Code Ann. § 70.24.015 (1996)** declares that STDs constitute an increasingly serious and sometimes fatal threat to the state's public welfare. Requires all programs designed to deal with STDs meet patient's privacy, confidentiality and dignity. Requires the state to make programs that meet emerging needs and operate efficiently and effectively, while reducing the incidence of STDs. Mandates all information be confidential.

WA   **Wash. Rev. Code Ann. § 70.24.022 (1996)** requires the board to adopt rules authorizing interviews of all persons infected with an STD, investigate the source, and the order to submit to an examination, counseling and treatment of an infected or believed to be infected person. Requires all information gathered to be confidential. Allows a person who is reasonably believed to be infected with an STD to reveal the name or names of sexual contacts and not be held liable. Makes it a gross misdemeanor for any person who knowingly gives any false information concerning the existence of any STD.

WA   **Wash. Rev. Code Ann. § 70.24.024 (1996)** authorizes state and local health officers or other authorized persons to examine any person believed to be infected or exposed to an STD. Authorizes a health officer to order a person to submit to a medical examination, testing, counseling or treatment within 14 days of the initial investigation. Authorizes a health officer to restrict a person from any behavior or conduct that endangers the public. Requires these restrictions be in writing. Outlines issuance of the restriction order and court proceedings. Requires all information be confidential unless a public hearing is requested.

WA   **Wash. Rev. Code Ann. § 70.24.034 (1996)** authorizes a health officer to bring action in superior court when all other efforts have failed to detain a person who is engaging in behaviors that present a danger to the public health. Outlines superior court procedure. Requires superior court hearing be closed and confidential unless a public hearing is requested.

WA   **Wash. Rev. Code Ann. § 70.24.105 (Supplemental 1997)** prohibits any person to disclose or be compelled to disclose the identity of any person who has investigated, considered or requested a test or treatment for an STD. Allows for the exchange of medical information with certain authorized medical and social services personnel, law enforcement officers or by court order. Allows disclosure of test results upon the request of a victim of a sex crime.

WA   **Wash. Rev. Code Ann. § 70.24.130 (1996)** authorizes the board to adopt rules to implement and enforce regulating STDs. Requires the rules to protect the confidentiality of persons investigated and records.

WV   **W. Va. Code § 16-4A-3 (1995)** requires a physician to test the blood of a pregnant woman for syphilis and indicate on the blood sample that the blood specimen is from a pregnant woman. Outlines reporting requirements and requires the results be reported to the state. Requires all laboratory results and reports of a syphilis test for a pregnant woman be confidential and not be open for public inspection.

WI   **Wis. Stat. Ann. § 252.10 (West Supplemental 1997)** requires reports, examinations and inspections and all records concerning STD, be confidential and not open to public inspection unless necessary for the safety of public health.

WI   **Wis. Stat. Ann. § 252.10 (West Supplemental 1997)** allows a health care professional to test an individual for STDs without first obtaining informed consent to do the testing. Prohibits disclosure of name of test subject on any sample used for performance of an STD test.

WY   **Wyo. Stat. § 7-1-109 (1977)** requires testing for STDs in sexual offense cases. Outlines court procedures. Requires examination results to be reported to the appropriate health officer. Requires the health officer to notify the victim, alleged victim or, if a minor, the parents or guardian of the victim or the alleged victim. Requires costs of any medical examination be funded through the department. Requires all results be held confidential and inadmissible as evidence in court and will remain undisclosed except under certain circumstances.

WY   **Wyo. Stat. § 35-4-132 (1997)** requires all STD information and records be confidential. Requires that no information be disclosed unless with written consent, for statistical purposes, or as a necessity for the administration and enforcement of controlling and treating STDs.

WY   **Wyo. Stat. § 35-4-133 (1997)** allows a health worker to request testing of a person who possibly is infected with an STD. Allows the county to apply for a court order to have a test performed if the patient does not consent to testing. Requires test results be kept confidential and reported to the state.

Consent—Release of Records

AL   **Ala. Code § 22-11A-22 (1997)** maintains that all records are confidential and cannot be used against the patient. Release of records is allowed only with the written consent of the patient. Makes it a Class C misdemeanor for medical records of infected persons to be released without written consent of the patient.

DE   **Del. Code Ann. tit. 16, § 712 (1996)** prohibits public health officials from disclosing any information about the records of a person infected or being treated for STDs or HIV without the consent of that person.

KS   **Kan. Stat. Ann § 65-153f (Supplemental 1997)** requires a physician or a person attending a pregnant woman, with the consent of the woman, to take a blood sample for a serological test for syphilis and Hepatitis B within 14 days after the diagnosis of pregnancy. Requires an approved laboratory report all positive or reactive tests. Requires all laboratory reports, files and records to be confidential and only be opened by authorized health officers or by written consent of the woman.

KY   **Ky. Rev. Stat. § 214.420 (1995)** declares confidentiality is essential for the proper control and prevention of STDs. Requires all information and reports regarding a person infected with or suspected of being infected with an STD be confidential. Specifies only authorized health department personnel who are assigned to STD control activities have access to records and reports. Allows for medical information to be released to the physician of a person suspected of being infected, for statistical purposes where the individual is not identified, with written consent from the person for the information to be released, and in case of a medical emergency.

MT   **Mont. Code Ann. § 41-1-403 (1997)** allows, but does not obligate, the physician to inform the spouse, parent or guardian of a minor receiving treatment for a venereal disease when severe complications are present or anticipated, major surgery or hospitalization is needed, the hospital desires a third-party commitment to pay for services, failure to inform the parent would jeopardize the safety of the minor or to inform them would benefit the minor's physical mental health. Prohibits information from being disclosed to the parent or guardian without the consent of the minor when the minor is found not to be pregnant, suffering from drug abuse or infected with an STD.

MT   **Mont. Code Ann. § 50-18-109 (1997)** outlines the release of information when permitted. Allows information concerning a person infected or suspected to be infected with an STD to be released only to authorized personnel of the department, to a physician who has written consent of the person whose record is requested, or to a local health officer engaged in the eradication of STDs. Specifies the importance to protecting and preserving the principle of confidentiality.

NV   **Nev. Rev. Stat. § 441A.230 (1993)** prohibits any person from disclosing the name or any identifying information without the consent of the person infected with the STD.

SC   **S.C. Code Ann. § 44-29-135 (Law. Co-op 1997)** requires information not be released or made public except with the written consent of persons identified. Allows information to be released for statistical purposes where the individual cannot be identified, and for medical information necessary to enforce the control and treatment of STDs and protect the health of the STD-infected person. Requires reporting the name and the medical information of a minor with no further information required to be released by the department.

WA   **Wash. Rev. Code Ann. § 70.24.105 (Supplemental 1997)** prohibits any person to disclose or be compelled to disclose the identity of any person who has investigated, considered or requested a test or treatment for an STD. Allows for the exchange of medical information with certain authorized medical and social services personnel, law enforcement officers or by court order. Allows disclosure of test results upon the request of a victim of a sex crime.

WY   **Wyo. Stat. § 35-4-132 (1997)** requires all STD information and records be confidential. Requires that no information be disclosed unless with written consent, for statistical purposes, or as a necessity for the administration and enforcement of controlling and treating STDs.

Counseling

AK   **Alaska Stat. § 18.15.310** requires that all blood drawn for a court-ordered HIV or STD test of a person charged with a sex offense be performed by a physician, physician's assistant or other qualified personnel and tested in a medically approved laboratory. Requires all test results that indicate exposure to or infection by HIV or other STDs be reported to the department. Requires anyone who receives test results, other than the test subjects, maintain confidentiality. Requires the department provide free counseling and free testing to the victim for HIV and other STDs and counseling to the alleged sex offender upon request of the offender. Requires the department to provide referral to appropriate health care facilities and support services at the request of the victim.

FL   **Fla. Stat. Ann. § 384.27 (West 1993 and Supplemental 1998)** outlines the procedures for physical examinations and treatment of STDs. Specifies that no person can be apprehended, examined or treated for STDs against his or her will, except upon court order. States that the suspected STD-infected person receive written notice within 72 hours of the court order requiring the person to receive treatment. Requires the department to provide clear and convincing evidence that a threat to public health exists when petitioning the court for an order. Allows the court to require counseling and periodic testing for the suspected STD-infected person.

IL   **Ill. Ann. Stat. ch. 410 § 70/5 (Smith-Hurd 1997)** requires minimum requirements for hospitals providing emergency services to sexual assault survivors. Hospitals must offer sexual assault survivors a blood test to determine the presence of an STD, written and oral instructions indicating the need for a second blood test six weeks after the sexual assault to determine the presence or absence of an STD, appropriate oral and written information about the possibility of infection of an STD and pregnancy resulting from the sexual assault, oral and written information about accepted medical procedures and medication available for the prevention or treatment of a venereal disease infection resulting from a sexual assault, and information to provide or refer the victim to counseling.

IL   **Ill. Ann. Stat. ch. 410 § 210/4 (Smith-Hurd 1997)** outlines the protocol for the treatment and care of minors for STDs, alcoholism and addiction. Allows a minor 12 years or older to give consent to medical care or counseling for STDs. Specifies that the consent of a parent or legal guardian is not necessary when diagnosing or treating STDs for a minor patient.

IL   **Ill. Ann. Stat. ch. 410 § 210/5 (Smith-Hurd 1997)** releases any physician, psychologist, social worker or other qualified person who provides diagnosis, treatment or counseling to a minor for an STD from the obligation to inform the parent or guardian, without the minor's consent, unless the action is necessary to protect the safety of the minor, family member or individual.

LA   **La. Rev. Stat. Ann § 15:535 (West 1992 and Supplemental)** authorizes the court to order an adjudicated delinquent or a person convicted of a sexual offense to submit to an STD or HIV test. Requires the procedure or test to be performed by a qualified physician who is required to report any positive result to the Department of Public Safety and Corrections. Requires notification of the test results to the victim or the parent regardless of the results.

MI   **Mich. Stat. Ann. § 14.15 (5119) (Law. Co-op 1995)** requires a marriage applicant be counseled by a physician or other authorized medical personnel on the transmission and prevention of venereal diseases and HIV infection. Requires a county clerk to distribute to each applicant educational materials prepared by the department about testing and counseling for a venereal diseases and HIV. Prohibits a county clerk from issuing a marriage license to an applicant who fails to present a certificate indicating the applicant has received counseling regarding the transmission and prevention of venereal diseases and HIV from a physician and has been offered or referred for venereal disease or HIV testing.

MI   **Mich. Stat. Ann. § 14.15 (5121) (Law. Co-op 1995)** makes it a misdemeanor for a county clerk to issue a marriage license to an individual who fails to present a certificate stating the applicant has received counseling about venereal diseases and HIV and has been offered venereal disease and HIV testing. Makes it a misdemeanor for any person who discloses the marriage license applicant has taken a venereal disease or HIV test and discloses the results of the tests except when required by law. Makes it a misdemeanor for a physician who knowingly and willfully makes a false statement in a certificate required for a marriage license.

MT   **Mont. Code Ann. § 41-1-402 (1997)** allows a minor to consent to prevention, diagnosis and treatment from a licensed physician for a pregnancy, drug abuse or a venereal disease. Requires the physician treating a minor for a venereal disease to refer the minor to counseling.

NV   **Nev. Rev. Stat. § 441A.320 (1993)** authorizes the health authority to test a person for STDs and HIV who is arrested for a sex offense crime. Requires the health authority to disclose the results to the victim or victim's parent or guardian if that person is a minor. Requires the health authority, at the request of the victim, provide an examination and counseling. Requires the court to order all expenses be paid by the offender.

NM **N. M. Stat. Ann. § 24-1-9.2 (1997)** allows for STD testing of persons formally charged with or for allegedly committing certain criminal sexual offenses. Allows the victim of a criminal sexual offense to petition the court to order that a test be performed on the offender when consent to perform a test on an offender cannot be obtained, provided that the same test is first performed on the victim of the alleged criminal offense. Allows the parent or legal guardian to petition the court when the victim is a minor. Outlines court procedures. Requires court order to state that the offender be tested within 10 days after the petition is filed by the victim or parent. Allows results be disclosed only to the offender and the victim or the victim's parent or legal guardian. Allows for counseling for both the alleged offender and the victim.

NM **N. M. Stat. Ann. § 24-1-9.3 (1997)** requires mandatory counseling for all patients with positive STD test results. Requires counseling include the meaning of the test results and the possible need for additional testing, the availability of appropriate health care and social support services, and the benefits of locating and counseling any individual the infected person may have exposed to the STD.

NC **N.C. Gen. Stat. § 15A-615 (1997)** allows testing a sex offender who has had an alleged sexual contact with any minor under 16 years of age for STDs including chlamydia, gonorrhea, Hepatitis B, herpes, HIV and syphilis. Allows the victim to petition the court for the offender to be tested. Requires the test results be reported to the local health director. Requires the victim and alleged offender be informed of the test results and be provided with counseling. Requires the results of the test not be admissible as evidence in any criminal proceeding.

OK **Okla. Stat. Ann. tit. 63, § 1-525 (1997)** requires all information—including the records and test results of an infected person charged with a sex offense—be confidential and only be disclosed by court order. Allows the victim of the crime to request the results of the examination and test results conducted on the offender. Requires the department to provide free testing to the alleged victim for any venereal or communicable disease when the offender tests positive for any tests. Requires that the testing of the victim be accompanied with pretest and post-test counseling. Requires the state board of health to rule and regulate procedural guidelines for testing sex offenders and releasing records containing the sex offender's test results. Requires the guidelines to respect the rights of the person arrested for the alleged sex offense and the victim of the alleged sex offense.

PR **P.R. Laws Ann. tit. 24, § 578 (1993)** requires providers to counsel, interview and investigate anyone suspected of having an STD infection.

RI **R.I. Gen. Laws § 23-1-36.1 (1996)** requires the director of health to prepare and submit to each marriage license clerk's office in each town a packet of health information, including information about STDs and an "AIDS testing and notification form." Requires that the form state that the department provides confidential free HIV tests, pre-test and post-test educational materials and post-test counseling for the HIV-positive person.

RI **R.I. Gen. Laws § 23-11-17 (1996)** requires a physician or health care provider to offer testing for HIV to any person suspected of having an STD. Requires any person who is offered an HIV test and counseling to be provided with an "AIDS testing and notification form," which the person is required to sign and date in acknowledgement of the offer. Requires the department be responsible for costs associated with performing and reporting the results of the HIV test. Requires all persons tested for HIV/AIDS to be provided with counseling.

SC **S.C. Code Ann. § 16-3-740 (Law. Co-op 1997)** requires testing of certain convicted offenders for Hepatitis B, STDs and HIV within 15 days of the conviction. Outlines court procedures. Requires the convicted offender or adjudicated juvenile offender to pay for the test unless the offender is indigent, then the tests will be paid for by the state. Requires the state to provide the victim and the convicted offender with counseling if any of the tests are positive.

SC **S.C. Code Ann. § 16-15-255 (Law. Co-op 1997)** requires testing of certain sex offenders for Hepatitis B, STDs and HIV. Outlines court procedures. Requires the convicted offender to pay for the test unless the offender is indigent, then the tests will be paid for by the state. Requires the state provide the victim and the convicted offender with counseling if any of the tests are positive.

WA **Wash. Rev. Code Ann. § 70.24.022 (1996)** requires the board to adopt rules authorizing interviews of all persons infected with an STD, investigate the source, and the order to submit to an examination, counseling and treatment of an infected or believed to be infected person. Requires all information gathered to be confidential. Allows a person who is reasonably believed to be infected with an STD to reveal the name or names of sexual contacts and not be held liable. Makes it a gross misdemeanor for any person who knowingly gives any false information concerning the existence of any STD.

WA **Wash. Rev. Code Ann. § 70.24.024 (1996)** authorizes state and local health officers or other authorized persons to examine any person believed to be infected or exposed to an STD. Authorizes a health officer to order a person to submit to a medical examination, testing, counseling or treatment within 14 days of the initial investigation. Authorizes a health officer to restrict a person from any behavior or conduct that endangers the public. Requires these restrictions be in writing. Outlines issuance of the restriction order and court proceedings. Requires all information be confidential unless a public hearing is requested.

WA **Wash. Rev. Code Ann. § 70.24.095 (1996)** requires a health care practitioner attending a pregnant woman or attending a drug treatment program participant who is seeking treatment of an STD to ensure that the patient receives AIDS counseling.

WY **Wyo. Stat. § 35-4-133 (1997)** authorizes a health officer to isolate and examine an STD-infected or suspected to be an infected individual. Requires the individual to submit to treatment at public expense. Allows providing STD education information and counseling for the STD-infected individual. Requires the health officer to notify any person who may have been exposed. Requires the health officer to investigate sources of STDs and cooperate with the proper law enforcement in enforcing the laws against prostitution.

Court Proceedings and Penalties

AL   **Ala. Code § 22-11A-14 (1997)** outlines reporting procedures for STDs. Requires a physician who diagnoses or treats STDs to report to the state or county health officer. Requires laboratories to report all positive or reactive STD tests. Requires all reports and documentation be confidential. Makes it a misdemeanor for violating any reporting rules with a penalty ranging from $100 to $500 upon conviction.

AL   **Ala. Code § 22-11A-15 (1997)** requires a syphilis examination for a marriage license. Authorizes the Board of Health to charge a reasonable fee for testing. Makes it a Class C misdemeanor for physicians, ministers and others who fail to comply with procedures. Waives requirements for an emergency situation and defines an emergency.

AL   **Ala. Code § 22-11A-21 (1997)** makes it a Class C misdemeanor to treat, prescribe or sell medicine to a person with an STD if not authorized by a licensed physician. Makes it a Class C misdemeanor to knowingly transmit an STD to another person.

AL   **Ala. Code § 22-11A-22 (1997)** maintains that all records are confidential and cannot be used against the patient. Release of records is allowed only with the written consent of the patient. Makes it a Class C misdemeanor for medical records of infected persons to be released without written consent of the patient.

AL   **Ala. Code § 22-11A-24 (1997)** allows a state or county health officer to petition a probate judge of the county to commit a person to the custody of the department for compulsory testing, for treatment or quarantine, when any person who is exposed to an STD or where reasonable evidence indicates exposure to an STD, refuses testing or treatment, or whose conduct indicates exposure to others.

AK   **Alaska Stat. § 18.15.180** requires a physician to take a blood sample for syphilis from a pregnant woman. Makes it a misdemeanor for any physician who does not take a blood sample for syphilis, punishable by a fine of a maximum of $500. Exempts physicians whose patients refuse testing.

AK   **Alaska Stat. § 18.15.300** allows the court to order a person charged with a sex offense to be tested for HIV or STDs. Allows an alleged victim, parent or guardian, or attorney to petition the court to order tests. Requires copies of the test results be provided to the charged sex offender, each requesting victim, or, if the victim is a minor, the parent or guardian.

AK   **Alaska Stat. § 18.15.310** requires that all blood drawn for a court-ordered HIV or STD test of a person charged with a sex offense be performed by a physician, physician's assistant or other qualified personnel and tested in a medically approved laboratory. Requires all test results that indicate exposure to or infection by HIV or other STDs be reported to the department. Requires anyone who receives test results, other than the test subjects, maintain confidentiality. Requires the department to provide free counseling and free testing to the victim for HIV and other STDs and counseling to the alleged sex offender upon request of the offender. Requires the department to provide referral to appropriate health care facilities and support services at the request of the victim.

AK   **Alaska Stat. § 18.15.320** requires the cost for testing a person charged with a sex offense for HIV and other STDs be paid by the department. Requires the court to order the person to pay for the tests if convicted of the sex offense charge.

AR   **Ark. Stat. Ann. § 20-16-506 (1991)** makes it a misdemeanor for any physician or laboratory to fail to report a venereal disease with a punishable fine of no less than $10 and no more than $20.

CA   **Cal. Health & Safety Code § 120590-605 (West 1996)** requires the county district attorney to prosecute any person accused of violating the investigation, rules and regulations of reporting or treating a person with STDs.

CA   **Cal. Health & Safety Code § 120595 (West 1996)** requires any physician, health officer, spouse or other person to testify in the prosecution of the violation of any rule, regulation or quarantine of an STD.

CA   **Cal. Health & Safety Code § 120600-05 (West 1996)** makes it a misdemeanor for any person who refuses to give information or fails to comply with any proper control measure or examination for STDs, who exposes or infects another person with an STD, or who is infected with a venereal disease, and is infectious, and knows they are infected, to marry or have sexual intercourse. Specifies religious exemptions.

CA   **Cal. Health & Safety Code § 120715 (West 1996)** makes it a misdemeanor for any licensed physician or surgeon who attends a pregnant or recently delivered woman and does not obtain a blood sample for syphilis. Stipulates the authorized person is not guilty if the test is refused by the patient.

CO   **Colo. Rev. Stat. § 25-4-204 (1990)** makes it a misdemeanor, with a fine of no more than $300, for any physician who does not take a blood sample from a pregnant woman and submit it for a syphilis test. Releases any physician whose patient refuses a syphilis test from being found guilty of a misdemeanor.

CO   **Colo. Rev. Stat. § 25-4-407 (1997)** makes it a misdemeanor for any person to violate any department rule or regulation in regard to venereal diseases, with a punishable fine of no more than $300, or imprisonment in the county jail for no more than 90 days, or both.

CT   **Conn. Gen. Stat. § 54-102a (1997)** allows a court to order persons charged with certain sexual offenses to submit to a venereal examination and HIV testing. Requires reporting the results to the department. Allows the court to order treatment if HIV or a venereal disease is found. Requires the examination or test be paid for by the department. Makes it a Class C misdemeanor for any person who fails to comply with any court-ordered testing or treatment.

DE   **Del. Code Ann. tit. 16, § 704 (1996)** establishes the procedure for the apprehension, commitment, treatment, quarantine and possible court hearings of an STD-infected person. Sets guidelines for anyone who refuses to comply. Allows the director of the Division of Public Health to petition the courts for an order to quarantine and treat an infected person. Outlines the procedures.

DE   **Del. Code Ann. tit. 16, § 705 (1996)** outlines emergency public health procedures for suspected or infected persons who refuse testing, examination or treatment and who present a threat to the public health. Allows the director of the Division of Public Health to ask the court for an injunction or to take the infected person into custody.

DE   **Del. Code Ann. tit. 16, § 711 (1996)** maintains confidentiality of records and information. Allows records to be released for statistical purposes when the person's identity is anonymous and with the consent of all persons identified when enforcing the rules of the department concerning the control and treatment of STDs, in case of a medical emergency, and during civil and criminal litigation. Outlines the procedures for releasing confidential information during court proceedings.

DE   **Del. Code Ann. tit. 16, § 713 (1996)** requires any person who violates any rule or regulation for STDs made by the Department of Health and Social Services be fined no less than $100 and no more than $1,000. Imposes fines of no less than $25 and no more than $200 on any person who does not report an STD. Specifies that each separate day of violation be considered separate penalty offenses.

DC   **D. C. Stat. Code Ann. § 30-121 (1997)** makes it unlawful for any person who knowingly divulges any information about a premarital syphilis blood test, misrepresents or falsifies any facts about a premarital syphilis blood test, issues a marriage license without having received the syphilis-free statement by a licensed physician or fails to comply with taking a required syphilis test for a marriage license. Makes it punishable with a fine of $250, or be imprisoned for no more than six months, or both.

FL   **Fla. Stat. Ann. § 384.24 (West 1998)** makes it a misdemeanor of the first degree for a person infected with an STD or HIV to engage in sexual acts with a nonconsenting person or a person who is not informed of the infection.

FL   **Fla. Stat. Ann. § 384.25 (West 1998)** requires any person who violates the reporting procedures or does not maintain confidentiality to be fined up to $500 for each offense. Requires the department to report each violation to the regulatory agency responsible for licensing health care professionals and laboratories.

FL   **Fla. Stat. Ann. § 384.27 (West 1993 and Supplemental 1998)** outlines the procedures for physical examinations and treatment of STDs. Specifies that no person can be apprehended, examined or treated for STDs against his or her will, except upon court order. States that the suspected STD-infected person receive written notice within 72 hours of the court order requiring the person to receive treatment. Requires the department to provide clear and convincing evidence that a threat to public health exists when petitioning the court for an order. Allows the court to require counseling and periodic testing for the suspected STD-infected person.

FL   **Fla. Stat. Ann. § 384.28 (West 1993 and Supplemental 1998)** requires specific protocol be followed when attempting hospitalization, placement and treatment for an STD-infected person who is considered a threat to the public health. Allows the department to petition a court order for the hospitalization and treatment of an infected person. Prohibits placing a person under age 18 into a hospital or in another health care facility where adults are hospitalized.

54

FL   **Fla. Stat. Ann. § 384.281 (West 1993 and Supplemental 1998)** provides the department with guidelines for prehearing detention for an STD-infected person who is considered a threat to public health. Outlines procedures for confining an infected person. Requires an infected person to have a bail hearing within 24 hours.

FL   **Fla. Stat. Ann. § 384.282 (West 1993 and Supplemental 1998)** requires all court decisions, orders, petitions and other formal documents be protected and confidential. Requires the name of an infected person be protected in court by providing a fake name. Requires any court proceeding where the true name was used be sealed.

FL   **Fla. Stat. Ann. § 384.283 (West 1993 and Supplemental 1998)** requires all notices, petitions, warrants and orders used in the examination, hospitalization and treatment of an STD-infected person be served by the sheriff to the infected person. Requires the sheriff of the county that the infected person resides in to take the infected person into custody and deliver him or her to the designated facility.

FL   **Fla. Stat. Ann. § 384.284 (West 1993)** requires the department to develop and supply all necessary forms to be used by the circuit court for ordering the physical examination, treatment and hospitalization of an STD-infected person.

FL   **Fla. Stat. Ann. § 385.285 (West 1993 and Supplemental 1998)** allows any infected person who is being examined, treated or isolated by court order to appeal to the court and requires immediate release. Outlines reasons a person may be released, including that the person no longer poses an immediate threat to the public safety.

FL   **Fla. Stat. Ann. § 384.287 (West 1998)** allows for an officer, firefighter or paramedic who may have been exposed to an STD in the line of duty to request testing of the person they were exposed to as well as be tested themselves. Allows for a court order if the suspected person does not volunteer for testing. States that results are exempt from confidentiality.

FL   **Fla. Stat. Ann. § 384.34 (West 1993 and Supplemental 1998)** makes it a misdemeanor of the first degree when any person infected with an STD or HIV engages in sexual acts with a nonconsenting person or a person who is not informed of the infection. Makes it a misdemeanor of the first degree to break confidentiality during an STD investigation. Makes it a misdemeanor of the second degree for any person found of guilty of giving false information about the existence of an STD. Requires that a person who violates the rules of the department regarding STDs be fined no more than $500 for each violation.

FL   **Fla. Stat. Ann. § 796.08 (West 1998)** requires a person already convicted of prostitution to be tested for HIV and STDs when arrested for prostitution. States the penalties for prostituting or soliciting another for prostitution while knowing of the infection and not informing the other person involved.

GA   **Ga. Code Ann. § 19-3-40 (1991)** requires a blood test for syphilis 30 days before a marriage license is issued. Allows for free testing if the applicant is unable to pay. Requires a physician's certificate stating whether the applicant is infected or not infected. Outlines the procedure for granting a marriage license when the test is positive and partners are aware of the test results. Any judge, applicant or physician who violates the law by making a false statement is guilty of a misdemeanor.

GA   **Ga. Code Ann. § 42-1-7 (1997)** requires any state or county correctional institution, or municipal or county detention facility to notify the law enforcement agency of the transporting of an inmate or patient infected with any venereal disease, HIV or other infectious, communicable disease. Requires information released for the transporting be kept confidential and only be released or obtained by the institution, facilities or agencies that are involved with the transporting of the infected patient or inmate. Makes it a misdemeanor for any person to make any unauthorized disclosure of the transporting information.

HI   **Hawaii Rev. Stat. § 325-53 (1993)** requires a report accompany the birth or death certificate that states a woman who gave birth to a child was tested for syphilis. States that failure to test or report for syphilis may be punishable up to a $1,000 fine per violation.

HI   **Hawaii Rev. Stat. § 325-54 (1993)** maintains confidentiality of reports and outlines the penalties for violating confidentiality. Requires any person breaking confidentiality be fined $500 or imprisoned for no more than 90 days or both.

HI   **Hawaii Rev. Stat. § 325-56 (1993)** mandates that a physician or other person permitted by law to attend to a pregnant woman, who does not take a blood sample for a syphilis test, does not report positive syphilis blood test or violates any rule of the department for testing syphilis be fined no more than $1,000 per violation. Authorizes the director of health to impose the penalties.

ID   **Idaho Code § 39-601 (1993)** defines venereal diseases as syphilis, gonorrhea, HIV/AIDS, AIDS related complexes (ARC), chancroid and Hepatitis B and are considered contagious, infectious, communicable and dangerous to public health. Makes it unlawful for anyone infected with a venereal disease to knowingly expose another person to the infection.

ID   **Idaho Code § 39-606 (1993)** requires all reports regarding venereal disease be confidential. Makes it a misdemeanor for any person who willfully or maliciously discloses the contents of any confidential public health record except under written authorization by the infected person who is on the record.

ID   **Idaho Code § 39-607 (1993)** makes it a misdemeanor for any person to violate any venereal disease rule or regulation. Makes it a misdemeanor for any person infected with syphilis, gonorrhea or chancroid to expose another person to the infection, States that both misdemeanors are punishable with a fine of no more than $300, or six months in prison, or both.

ID   **Idaho Code § 39-1006 (1993)** states that any authorized medical person who does not request a syphilis test on a pregnant woman or a woman who recently delivered be found guilty of a misdemeanor. Stipulates that if testing is refused by the patient, the authorized person requesting the test not be found guilty of a misdemeanor.

IL   **Ill. Ann. Stat. ch. 410 § 325/4 (Smith-Hurd 1997)** outlines the reporting procedures for STDs. Requires any physician who diagnoses or treats STDs to report to the state or county health officer. Requires any laboratory that conducts STD testing report all positive or reactive tests. Makes it a Class A misdemeanor for any person who provides false information. Imposes $500 fines on any person who violates the rules of the department. Requires the department to report each violation to the regulatory agency responsible for licensing a health care professional or a laboratory.

IL   **Ill. Ann. Stat. ch. 410 § 325/5 (Smith-Hurd 1997)** requires the department to adopt rules regarding the authorization of interviews for investigating persons infected or believed to be infected with an STD, and to order a person to submit to an examination and treatment. Requires all information gathered during an investigation be confidential. Makes it a Class A misdemeanor for any person who knowingly discloses any information of any person infected with an STD.

IL   **Ill. Ann. Stat. ch. 410 § 325/6 (Smith-Hurd 1997)** authorizes the department to examine any person believed to be infected with an STD. Requires any person believed to be infected with an STD to submit to treatment. Prohibits any person from being apprehended, examined or treated for an STD without a warrant.

IL   **Ill. Ann. Stat. ch. 410 § 325/7 (Smith-Hurd 1997)** authorizes the department to quarantine and isolate any person suspected of being infected with an STD when they are a danger to the public health. States that no person may be quarantined or ordered into isolation except with the consent of the person or by court order.

IN   **Ind. Code Ann. § 16-41-14-15 (Burns 1993)** prohibits any person from disclosing or being compelled to disclose information collected for artificial insemination. Mandates that information may not be released or made public on subpoena except under certain circumstances. Lists exemptions.

IN   **Ind. Code Ann. § 16-41-14-16 (Burns 1993)** makes it a Class A misdemeanor for a practitioner who is responsible for conducting an STD screening test required for artificial insemination to knowingly or intentionally fail to conduct the screening test.

IN   **Ind. Code Ann. § 16-41-14-19 (Burns 1993)** allows the department to issue a civil penalty not to exceed $1,000 per violation per day against any person who fails to comply with the rules or the law governing the STD-testing of semen used in artificial insemination. Allows the department to bring action against a licensed facility for failing to test semen used in artificial insemination.

IN   **Ind. Code Ann. § 16-41-14-20 (Burns 1993)** makes it a Class B misdemeanor for a person who recklessly fails to comply or interferes with the inspection or investigation of an STD case. Constitutes a separate offense for each day a violation continues.

IA   **Iowa Code § 140.6 (1997)** makes it a simple misdemeanor for any physician or other person who is required to report a venereal disease who does not report or falsely reports any information concerning an STD-infected person, or who discloses the identity of that person. Requires that failure to report a venereal disease as specified may result in the refusal of a license renewal.

IA   **Iowa Code § 140.8 (1997)** authorizes the local board of health to examine any person reasonably suspected of having a venereal disease in an infectious state. Allows the local board to apply to the court for an order for that person to submit to venereal disease examination. Requires that in every case of treatment ordered by the court, a doctor must certify that the person no longer is infectious.

56

IA   **Iowa Code § 140.15 (1997)** makes it a simple misdemeanor for a person to violate any venereal disease control law.

KY   **Ky. Rev. Stat. § 214.990 (1995)** makes it unlawful for any physician who fails to take a blood sample from a pregnant woman and submit the sample for a syphilis test. Makes it unlawful for anyone who does not report any positive test results of a pregnant woman's syphilis test.

KY   **Ky. Rev. Stat. § 529.090 (1996)** makes it a Class A misdemeanor for any person who commits prostitution when he or she tested positive for an STD and could possibly infect another person through sexual activity.

LA   **La. Rev. Stat. Ann § 1062 (West 1992)** makes it unlawful for any person to infect or expose another person to a venereal disease.

LA   **La. Rev. Stat. Ann § 1066 (West 1992)** makes it unlawful for a person to sell any drug for the treatment of a venereal disease unless prescribed by a licensed physician.

LA   **La. Rev. Stat. Ann § 1068 (West 1992)** requires any person who violates any venereal disease rule or regulation on the first offense be fined no less than $10 and no more than $200.

LA   **La. Criminal Procedure Ann. art. 499 (West Supplemental)** requires a person charged by a grand jury for a sexual offense to undergo a medical procedure or tests for STDs and HIV/AIDS. Allows the court to provide the results of the test to the victim and the health authorities. Prohibits the state from using the fact that the test was performed on the alleged offender and the test results in any criminal proceedings arising out of the alleged offense.

MA   **Mass. Gen. Laws Ann. ch. 111, § 119 (West 1996)** requires morbidity reports and records pertaining to a venereal disease from hospitals and laboratories not be public record and the contents not to be divulged by any person having access, except under court order or to an authorized person. Makes it a violation for the first offense and punishable by a fine of no more than $50, and each subsequent offense by a fine of no more than $100.

MI   **Mich. Stat. Ann. § 14.15 (5121) (Law. Co-op 1995)** makes it a misdemeanor for a county clerk to issue a marriage license to an individual who fails to present a certificate stating the applicant has received counseling about venereal diseases and HIV and has been offered venereal disease and HIV testing. Makes it a misdemeanor for any person who discloses the marriage license applicant has taken a venereal disease or HIV test and discloses the results of the tests except when required by law. Makes it a misdemeanor for a physician who knowingly and willfully makes a false statement in a certificate required for a marriage license.

MI   **Mich. Stat. Ann. § 14.15 (5131) (Law. Co-op 1995)** requires all reports, records and data pertaining to the testing, treatment, reporting and research of venereal diseases, HIV/AIDS and other serious communicable diseases be confidential. Makes it a misdemeanor for any person who violates confidentiality, which is punishable by imprisonment of no more than one year, or a fine of not more than $5,000, or both.

MS   **Miss. Code Ann. § 41-23-27 (1993)** authorizes the state Board of Health to isolate, quarantine and treat a person infected with an STD. Authorizes the board to pass rules and regulations regarding isolation, quarantine, confinement and treatment. Makes it a misdemeanor for any person violating any rule or regulation made by the state Board of Health punishable by a fine, imprisonment or both.

MS   **Miss. Code Ann. § 41-23-29 (1993)** requires any person suspected of being infected with an STD be subject to an examination and inspection by the state Board of Health. Failure or refusal to be examined may be a misdemeanor.

MS   **Miss. Code Ann. § 99-37-25 (Supplement 1997)** requires the county pay for the STD tests and medical examination of an alleged sex offender. Requires the test results be made available to the victim or to the parent or guardian of the victim if the victim is a child. Requires any defendant who is convicted of rape, sexual battery of a child, touching or handling of a child or exploiting a child pay the county for the STD tests and medical examination.

MO   **Mo. Ann. Stat. § 210.060 (Vernon 1996)** makes it a misdemeanor for any licensed physician, midwife, registered nurse or other person who provides health care to a pregnant woman and who misrepresents the facts required for reporting any positive blood tests for syphilis or Hepatitis B. Requires that the crime be punishable by imprisonment of no more than a year, or by a fine of no more than $1,000, or both.

MT   **Mont. Code Ann. § 50-18-110 (1997)** makes it unlawful to prescribe, sell, or recommend any drugs, medicines or other substances for the cure or alleviation of a STD except by a prescription signed by a legally authorized person.

MT   **Mont. Code Ann. § 50-18-111 (1997)** allows a physician or health officer to issue a statement of freedom from diseases in an infectious state only if it is written in such a form or given under safeguards that will prevent its use in solicitation for sexual intercourse.

MT   **Mont. Code Ann. § 50-18-112 (1997)** makes it a misdemeanor for a person infected with an STD to knowingly expose another person to infection.

MT   **Mont. Code Ann. § 50-18-113 (1997)** makes it a misdemeanor for any person who violates the law or rules adopted by the department concerning an STD or who refuses to obey any lawful order issued by a state or local health officer.

MT   **Mont. Code Ann. § 50-19-103 (1997)** requires every female, regardless of age or marital status, seeking prenatal care from a physician, to submit a blood specimen for a standard serological test for syphilis. Requires the physician or an authorized person who attends a pregnant woman to take a blood sample at the first professional visit and submit it to a laboratory. Requires the physician designate it as a prenatal test when submitting. Penalizes any physician or authorized person required to take the blood sample who violates this statute with a misdemeanor. Exempts any physician or authorized person who requests a sample and is refused by the patient.

NE   **Neb. Rev. Stat. § 71-506 (1996)** makes it a Class V misdemeanor for any person who violates any STD rule or regulation of the department. Makes it a Class III misdemeanor for any person who willfully or maliciously breaks confidentiality and discloses the contents of any report, notification or investigation of an STD.

NV   **Nev. Rev. Stat. § 441A.320 (1993)** authorizes the health authority to test a person for STDs and HIV who is arrested for a sex offense crime. Requires the health authority to disclose the results to the victim or victim's parent or guardian if that person is a minor. Requires the health authority, at the request of the victim to provide an examination and counseling. Requires the court to order all expenses be paid by the offender.

NJ   **N.J. Stat. Ann. § 26:4-37 (West 1996)** allows a health officer, state commissioner of health or authorized representative to file a complaint with the court when a venereal disease-infected person fails or refuses to comply with a quarantine.

NJ   **N.J. Stat. Ann. § 26:4-49.7 (West 1996)** requires the court to order a person suspected of being infected with a venereal disease coming before the court on any charge to submit to an examination and treatment.

NM   **N. M. Stat. Ann. § 24-1-9.1 (1997)** allows for STD testing of persons convicted of certain criminal offenses. Allows the victim of a criminal sexual offense to petition the court to order a test be performed on the offender when a consent to perform a test cannot be obtained. Allows the parent or legal guardian to petition the court when the victim is a minor. Requires the court order to state that the test be administered to the offender within 10 days after the petition is filed. Requires the test results be disclosed only to the offender and the victim or the victim's parent or legal guardian.

NM   **N. M. Stat. Ann. § 24-1-9.2 (1997)** allows for STD testing of persons formally charged with or allegedly committing certain criminal sexual offenses. Allows the victim of a criminal sexual offense to petition the court to order that a test be performed on the offender when consent to perform a test on an offender cannot be obtained, provided that the same test is first performed on the victim of the alleged criminal offense. Allows the parent or legal guardian to petition the court when the victim is a minor. Outlines court procedures. Requires court order to state that the offender be tested within 10 days after the petition is filed by the victim or parent. Allows results be disclosed only to the offender and the victim or the victim's parent or legal guardian. Allows for counseling for both the alleged offender and the victim.

NM   **N. M. Stat. Ann. § 24-1-9.5 (1997)** prohibits any person who sees the results of an STD test to disclose the test results to another person, except as authorized. Requires that whenever disclosure is made it is accompanied by a statement stating the disclosure policy and the penalty of a petty misdemeanor for disclosing.

NM   **N. M. Stat. Ann. § 24-1-9.7 (1997)** mandates that any person who makes an unauthorized disclosure of confidential information be found guilty of a petty misdemeanor and sentenced to imprisonment in the county jail for a maximum of six months, or payment of a fine of not more than $500, or both.

NM   **N. M. Stat. Ann. § 30-9-5 (1994)** allows the court to order a venereal disease examination and treatment for a person convicted of prostitution or soliciting a prostitute. Requires the state to pay for medical treatment when the infected person is unable to pay.

58

NY   **N.Y. Public Health Law § 2301 (McKinney 1993)** allows a health officer to apply to court for an order to examine a person who is refusing to be tested for an STD. Requires all papers pertaining to any proceedings be kept confidential except to those authorized to inspect the report.

NY   **N.Y. Public Health Law § 2302 (McKinney 1993)** requires any person arrested for failure to comply with a court order for an STD examination or arrested for frequenting houses of prostitution be examined for STDs. Outlines court procedures. Prohibits the release of any person convicted until that person has been examined.

NY   **N.Y. Public Health Law § 2306 (McKinney 1993)** requires all STD reports and information be confidential. Allows for information to be disclosed by court order in certain criminal proceedings provided that the subject of the information has waived confidentiality. Allows parents or guardians of minors to waive confidentiality.

NY   **N.Y. Public Health Law § 2307 (McKinney 1993)** makes it a misdemeanor when any person who knowingly is infected with an STD and has sexual intercourse with another person.

NY   **N.Y. Public Health Law § 2309 (McKinney 1993)** makes it a misdemeanor when or any person who violates the rules and regulations of the department regarding testing, reporting and confidentiality of STDs.

ND   **N.D. Cent. Code § 23-07-21 (1997)** makes it unlawful for anyone infected with an STD to willfully expose and infect another with the infection.

ND   **N.D. Cent. Code § 23-07.7-01 (1997)** allows the court to order any defendant or any alleged juvenile offender charged with a sex offense to submit to medical testing for STDs. Allows the court to order the testing only if the court receives a petition from the alleged victim. Requires a copy of the test results be released to the defendant's or alleged juvenile offender's physician and each requesting victim's physician. Outlines court procedures.

ND   **N.D. Cent. Code § 23-07.7-02 (1997)** outlines testing procedures for court-ordered testing. Requires testing for HIV and STDs. Requires laboratory to send a copy of test results to the physician who supplies results to defendant and victim, and the department. Makes it a Class C felony for any person who violates confidentiality.

OH   **Ohio Rev. Code Ann. § 2907.27 (Page 1996)** requires any person charged with rape, sexual battery, corruption of a minor, solicitation, solicitation after being found HIV positive, prostitution and prostitution after being found HIV positive, to be tested for a venereal disease upon request of the victim. Requires the accused to submit to medical treatment if found to be suffering from a venereal disease in an infectious stage. Requires the cost of the medical treatment be paid by the accused. Requires the court to order the accused to report for treatment at a health facility operated by the city if the accused is unable to pay.

OK   **Okla. Stat. Ann. tit. 21, § 1192 (1982 and Supplemental 1998)** makes it a felony for anyone to infect another with syphilis, gonorrhea or any other infectious disease.

OK   **Okla. Stat. Ann. tit. 43, § 32 (1990)** outlines the procedure for a judge ordering an extension of no more than 90 days for using a doctor's certificate stating that a premarital exam for syphilis was completed for a marriage license. Requires the judge to be satisfied that both parties are of no harm to society.

OK   **Okla. Stat. Ann. tit. 43, § 37 (1990)** makes it a misdemeanor for any marriage license applicant, physician, governmental or laboratory representative to misrepresent any facts or break confidentiality about any syphilis record or lab report.

OK   **Okla. Stat. Ann. tit. 63, § 1-518 (1997)** makes it unlawful for any STD-infected person to refuse, fail or neglect to report to an examination and treatment by a physician.

OK   **Okla. Stat. Ann. tit. 63, § 1-519 (1997)** makes it a felony for an infected person, before being discharged and pronounced cured in writing by a physician, to marry or to expose any person to a venereal disease.

OK   **Okla. Stat. Ann. tit. 63, § 1-520 (1997)** makes it a misdemeanor for any physician who discharges an STD-infected person early from treatment or provides a written statement stating an infected person is noninfectious.

OK   **Okla. Stat. Ann. tit. 63, § 1-521 (1997)** makes it unlawful for any person who is not a physician to treat an STD-infected person for pay unless acting under the direction of a physician.

OK   **Okla. Stat. Ann. tit. 63, § 1-522 (1997)** makes it unlawful for any person to offer or provide treatment, sell or furnish any medication to an STD-infected person without a prescription.

OK   **Okla. Stat. Ann. tit. 63, § 1-524 (1997)** requires examining all prisoners to determine if a prisoner is infected with an STD. Allows a licensed physician to examine persons who are arrested for prostitution or other sex crimes. Allows for a person to be detained until the results are known. Requires any person found to be infected with an STD to be treated. Requires quarantining any person who refuses treatment. Requires a person who is arrested for rape and other serious sexual crimes be tested for STDs and HIV. Authorizes the court to issue an order for testing during the arraignment. Requires the order not to include the name and address of the alleged victim. Requires the alleged victim be notified of the test results.

OK   **Okla. Stat. Ann. tit. 63, § 1-525 (1997)** requires all information including the records and test results of an infected person charged with a sex offense be confidential and only be disclosed by court order. Allows the victim of the crime to request the results of the examination and test results conducted on the offender. Requires the department to provide free testing to the alleged victim for any venereal or communicable disease when the offender tests positive for any tests. Requires testing of the victim be accompanied with pretest and post-test counseling. Requires the state board of health to rule and regulate procedural guidelines for testing sex offenders and releasing records containing the sex offender's test results. Requires the guidelines to respect the rights of the person arrested for the alleged sex offense and the victim of the alleged sex offense.

OK   **Okla. Stat. Ann. tit. 63, § 1-531 (1997)** makes it unlawful for any physician or health officer to issue a certificate stating that person is free from venereal disease except authorized by law, rule or regulation.

PA   **Pa. Cons. Stat. Ann. tit. 35, § 521.8 (Purdon 1993)** authorizes a local health officer to require any person suspected of being infected with a venereal disease to be examined and treated. Allows the health officer to quarantine any person who refuses treatment. Allows the health officer to file a court petition stating the person is suspected of being infected with a venereal disease.

PA   **Pa. Cons. Stat. Ann. tit. 35, § 521.8 (Purdon 1993)** allows any person taken into custody and charged with a sex offense crime to be examined for a venereal disease by a department or court-appointed physician. Allows any person convicted of a crime and suspected of being infected to be examined for a venereal disease. Requires treating any person found to be infected with a venereal disease.

PA   **Pa. Cons. Stat. Ann. tit. 35, § 521.8 (Purdon 1993)** authorizes a local health officer to require any person suspected of being infected with a venereal disease to be examined and treated. Allows the health officer to quarantine any person who refuses treatment. Allows the health officer to file a court petition stating the person is suspected of being infected with a venereal disease.

PA   **Pa. Cons. Stat. Ann. tit. 35, § 521.11 (Purdon 1993)** allows any local health officer to quarantine any person infected with a venereal disease who refuses treatment. Allows the secretary or local health officer to file a court petition to commit the infected person to the appropriate institution or hospital. Allows for the religious treatment as long as the quarantine requirement is kept. Allows the department to use any county jail for isolating the infected person during treatment. Requires the local board or department to reimburse the institution for use of treating the infected person.

PA   **Pa. Cons. Stat. Ann. tit. 35, § 521.12 (Purdon 1993)** makes it unlawful for a physician or representative from a laboratory to misrepresent any facts regarding a premarital examination for syphilis.

PR   **P.R. Laws Ann. tit. 24, § 575b (1993)** provides that STD test results are inadmissable in court proceedings as evidence, except when authorized by the individual.

PR   **P.R. Laws Ann. tit. 24, § 583 (1993)** outlines penalties for anyone who violates the laws as they relate to STDs. States penalties of up to six months in jail and fines up to $500 upon conviction.

RI   **R.I. Gen. Laws § 23-11-1 (1996)** makes it unlawful for anyone knowingly to expose another person to an STD. Requires any person found guilty to be fined no more than $100, or imprisoned for no more than three months.

RI   **R.I. Gen. Laws § 23-11-7 (1996)** requires a penalty for failure to report an STD case. Requires any superintendent, physician or other who fails to report an STD case within a 10-day period of first knowing about the case be fined no more than $100.

RI   **R.I. Gen. Laws § 23-11-8 (1996)** requires a physician to obtain a blood specimen from a pregnant woman within 30 days after the first professional visit. Requires the blood specimen be submitted to the state laboratory or to an approved laboratory for a standard test for syphilis. Makes it a misdemeanor for failing to take a sample and requires a fine of no less than $10 and no more than $100.

RI   **R.I. Gen. Laws § 23-11-9 (1996)** requires all records be confidential. Requires that any person who divulges the name of or gives any information relating to a person suffering from an STD be imprisoned for no more than six months or fined no more than $250.

RI **R.I. Gen. Laws § 23-11-12 (1996)** makes it a misdemeanor for any person who refuses an examination for STDs and upon conviction be punished by a $50 fine, or by imprisonment for 30 days, or both.

RI **R.I. Gen. Laws § 23-11-16 (1996)** penalizes, upon conviction, any person who violates any rule or regulation regarding STDs adopted by the department, by imposing a fine of no more than $100, or by imprisonment for not more than 30 days, or both.

SC **S.C. Code Ann. § 16-3-740 (Law. Co-op 1997)** requires testing of certain convicted offenders for Hepatitis B, STDs and HIV within 15 days of the conviction. Outlines court procedures. Requires the convicted offender or adjudicated juvenile offender to pay for the test unless the offender is indigent, then the tests will be paid for by the state. Requires the state to provide the victim and the convicted offender with counseling if any of the tests are positive.

SC **S.C. Code Ann. § 44-29-60 (Law. Co-op 1997)** declares that STDs are contagious, infectious, communicable and dangerous to public health. Makes it a misdemeanor for anyone infected with STDs to knowingly expose another to infection.

SC **S.C. Code Ann. § 44-29-120 (Law. Co-op 1985)** requires a physician to take a blood sample of a pregnant woman within three days after her first examination and submit the sample to an approved laboratory for a standard serological test for syphilis, rubella and Rh factor. Requires other persons allowed to attend a pregnant woman but not allowed to take a blood sample make sure the sample is taken. Makes it a misdemeanor, punishable by a fine of no more than $100 and imprisonment for no more than 30 days, for anyone who does not take a sample for a syphilis test. Allows for religious exemption.

SD **S.D. Codified Laws Ann. § 34-23-1 (1994)** defines syphilis, gonorrhea and chancroid as venereal diseases that are contagious, infectious, communicable and dangerous to public health. Makes it a Class 2 misdemeanor for anyone infected with a venereal disease to expose another person to the infection.

SD **S.D. Codified Laws Ann. § 34-23-14 (1994)** makes it a Class 1 misdemeanor for any person who violates any rule or regulation for venereal diseases or any person who refuses to obey any order issued by a state, county or municipal health officer.

SD **S.D. Codified Laws Ann. § 34-23-18 (1994)** requires that any hospital, public clinic or licensed physician who provides the diagnosis, care or treatment of a venereal disease to a minor not incur any civil or criminal liability. Requires that immunity not apply to any negligent acts or omissions.

TN **Tenn. Code Ann. § 68-10-107 (1996)** prohibits any person infected with an STD to expose another person to such infection.

TN **Tenn. Code Ann. § 68-10-110 (1996)** allows a health officer to appeal to the court for an arrest of a person infected with an STD who refuses treatment. Outlines court procedures for the arrest and temporary commitment for treatment. Requires the examination be made by a health officer or licensed and practicing physician. Allows the infected person to have his or her own physician present at the exam. Allows for an appeal by the infected person.

TN **Tenn. Code Ann. § 68-10-111 (1996)** makes it a Class C misdemeanor for any health officer or any person who fails to perform the duties required of them by STD rule or bylaw or who violates any STD rule or bylaw.

TN **Tenn. Code Ann. § 68-10-113 (1996)** requires all records of information held by the department relating to known or suspected cases of STDs be confidential. Requires such information not be released or placed in court documents except under certain circumstances. Requires, under the Tennessee Child Abuse Law, reporting any STD case involving a minor younger than age 13 to the appropriate authorities.

TN **Tenn. Code Ann. § 68-10-114 (1996)** requires than no state or local department officer be asked in civil, criminal or other proceeding about the existence or contents of pertinent records of a person examined or treated for an STD.

TX **Tex. Family Code Ann § 54.033 (Vernon 1996)** outlines juvenile justice proceedings for STD and HIV testing. Requires a juvenile found delinquent of certain crimes to undergo an STD and HIV/AIDS test at the direction of the court or at the request of the victim. Allows the court to order a test if the child refuses to consent to the procedure or test. Prohibits the court from releasing the test result to anyone other than an authorized person.

VT **Vt. Stat. Ann. tit. 18, § 1092 (1982)** requires any physician or other qualified person providing medical care to a person infected with gonorrhea or syphilis to report the case to the state. Requires the infected person submit to treatment until discharged by a physician. Stipulates that any person who refuses treatment be reported to the state and punished by a fine of no more than $100, or three months in prison, or both.

VT   **Vt. Stat. Ann. tit. 18, § 1094 (1982)** allows any person suspected of being infected with a venereal disease to petition the court so that no examination or tests be made. Requires the petition not be a public record. Requires the suspected person be informed of the right to petition.

VT   **Vt. Stat. Ann. tit. 18, § 1096 (1982)** makes it a violation for any person infected with a venereal disease to refuse treatment, with a fine of no more than $500, or be imprisonment for no more than six months, or both.

VT   **Vt. Stat. Ann. tit. 18, § 1105 (1982)** makes it a crime for a person infected with gonorrhea or syphilis to marry while the disease is in a communicable stage. Makes the crime punishable by imprisonment for no less than two years, or a fine of no less than $500, or both.

VT   **Vt. Stat. Ann. tit. 18, § 1106 (1982)** makes it a crime for a person who knowingly is infected with gonorrhea or syphilis to have sex with another person, punishable for up to two years in prison, or a fine of no more than $500, or both.

VT   **Vt. Stat. Ann. tit. 13, § 2634 (1974)** requires medical treatment be given to a person convicted of prostitution and infected with a venereal disease before probation or parole to prevent the spread of such disease.

VA   **Va. Code § 32. 1-57 (1997)** allows a local health director to require any person suspected of being infected with any venereal disease to submit to an examination, testing and treatment. Allows the local health director to apply to the court for any order if the person refuses to submit to an examination, testing or treatment or fails to continue treatment. Requires treatment be free of charge when an infected person with a venereal disease is required by the local health director to receive treatment.

VA   **Va. Code § 32. 1-73 (1997)** makes it punishable, with the penalty of losing their license, for any physician, nurse or midwife who fails to comply with testing a pregnant woman for venereal diseases.

WA   **Wash. Rev. Code Ann. § 70.24.022 (1996)** requires the board to adopt rules authorizing interviews of all persons infected with an STD, to investigate the source and to order an infected or believed to be infected person to submit to an examination, counseling and treatment. Requires all information gathered to be confidential. Allows a person who is reasonably believed to be infected with an STD to reveal the name or names of sexual contacts and not be held liable. Makes it a gross misdemeanor for any person who knowingly gives any false information concerning the existence of any STD.

WA   **Wash. Rev. Code Ann. § 70.24.024 (1996)** authorizes state and local health officers or other authorized persons to examine any person believed to be infected or exposed to an STD. Authorizes a health officer to order a person to submit to a medical examination, testing, counseling or treatment within 14 days of the initial investigation. Authorizes a health officer to restrict a person from any behavior or conduct that endangers the public. Requires these restrictions be in writing. Outlines issuance of the restriction order and court proceedings. Requires all information be confidential unless a public hearing is requested.

WA   **Wash. Rev. Code Ann. § 70.24.034 (1996)** authorizes a health officer to bring action in superior court when all other efforts have failed to detain a person engaging in behaviors that present a danger to the public health. Outlines superior court procedure. Requires superior court hearing be closed and confidential unless a public hearing is requested.

WA   **Wash. Rev. Code Ann. § 70.24.080 (1996)** makes it a gross misdemeanor for any person who violates any provision or any lawful rule regarding STDs or HIV adopted by the board or who fails or refuses to obey any lawful order issued by any state or county municipal health officer.

WA   **Wash. Rev. Code Ann. § 70.24.140 (1996)** makes it unlawful for a person who has an STD to have sex unless the partner of the infected person has been informed.

WA   **Wash. Rev. Code Ann. § 70.24.150 (1996)** provides immunity from civil action for state and local boards of health members, public health officers, and employees of the department for damages arising from the performance of their duties in regulating STDs, unless in gross negligence.

WV   **W. Va. Code § 16-4-7 (1995)** makes it a misdemeanor for any physician or other person required to make a venereal disease report to fail to report or to make false statements on the report. Allows the medical licensing board to revoke the license of a physician for failing to give or provide false information about a person with a venereal disease.

WV   **W. Va. Code § 16-4-9 (1995)** requires a physician or other person who examines or treats a person with syphilis, gonorrhea or chancroid to inform that person of the necessity of taking treatment and continuing the treatment as prescribed. Requires a physician to report a patient who has stopped treatment to the local health officer. Makes it a misdemeanor for anyone to stop treatment for a venereal disease. Requires the local health officer to investigate any unfinished treatments for a venereal disease. Authorizes the local health officer to arrest, detain, and quarantine any patient who fails to return for treatment.

WV   **W. Va. Code § 16-4-18 (1995)** makes it unlawful for any person having a venereal disease in an infectious stage to work at a barber shop, bakery, hotel or restaurant. Requires the physician reporting the venereal disease case to notify the local health officer about the employee. Makes it a misdemeanor for anyone who is infected with a venereal disease who does not stop working within 24 hours.

WV   **W. Va. Code § 16-4-20 (1995)** makes it unlawful for any person suffering from an infectious venereal disease to expose another person to the infection. Requires a physician not to give a certificate stating the infected person is free from a venereal disease but to state the results of the examination and tests.

WV   **W. Va. Code § 16-4-21 (1995)** authorizes a health officer to establish a quarantine for a person infected with a venereal disease. Makes it a misdemeanor for anyone who does not follow the health officer's quarantining rules.

WV   **W. Va. Code § 16-4-24 (1995)** makes it a misdemeanor for a druggist or other person who is not a licensed physician to prescribe, recommend or sell any medicine to be used for treating syphilis, gonorrhea or chancroid.

WV   **W. Va. Code § 16-4A-5 (1995)** makes it a misdemeanor for any physician or laboratory to knowingly misrepresent any facts regarding testing on any laboratory report or birth or stillbirth certificate.

WI   **Wis. Stat. Ann. § 252.10 (West Supplemental 1997)** requires a physician to notify the department when an STD-infected person refuses or stops treatment. Authorizes the department to take the necessary steps to have the person committed for treatment or observation. Allows the court to commit to treatment persons who refuse. Outlines court procedures.

WY   **Wyo. Stat. § 35-4-130 (1997)** makes it a misdemeanor for any person violating or refusing to comply with the rules and regulations regarding STD testing, treatment and reporting, punishable by a fine of no more than $750, imprisonment for no more than six months, or both.

WY   **Wyo. Stat. § 35-4-133 (1997)** allows a health worker to request testing of a person possibly infected with an STD. Allows the county to apply for a court order to have a test performed if the patient does not consent to testing. Requires test results be kept confidential and reported to the state.

WY   **Wyo. Stat. § 35-4-504 (1997)** makes it a misdemeanor with a fine of no more than $100 for any doctor who does not take a blood sample from a pregnant woman for a syphilis test. States that any doctor who is refused by the pregnant patient to submit to a blood sample be found guilty of a misdemeanor.

WY   **Wyo. Stat. § 7-1-109 (1977)** requires testing for STDs in sexual offense cases. Outlines court procedures. Requires examination results be reported to the appropriate health officer. Requires the health officer to notify the victim, alleged victim or, if a minor, the parents or guardian of the victim or the alleged victim. Requires costs of any medical examination be funded through the department. Requires all results be held confidential and are inadmissible as evidence in court and will remain undisclosed except under certain circumstances.

Criminal Exposure

CA   **Cal. Health & Safety Code § 120600-05 (West 1996)** makes it a misdemeanor for any person who refuses to give information or fails to comply with any proper control measure or examination for STDs, exposes to or infects another person with an STD, or for any person infected with a venereal disease who is infectious, and knows they are infected, to marry or have sexual intercourse. Specifies religious exemptions.

FL   **Fla. Stat. Ann. § 796.08 (West 1998)** requires a person already convicted of prostitution to be tested for HIV and STDs when arrested for prostitution. States the penalties for prostituting or soliciting another for prostitution while knowing of the infection and not informing the other person involved.

ID   **Idaho Code § 39-601 (1993)** defines "venereal diseases" as syphilis, gonorrhea, HIV/AIDS, AIDS related complexes (ARC), chancroid and Hepatitis B and are considered contagious, infectious, communicable and dangerous to public health. Makes it unlawful for anyone infected with a venereal disease to knowingly expose another person to the infection.

KY   **Ky. Rev. Stat. § 529.090 (1996)** makes it a Class A misdemeanor for any person who commits prostitution when he or she tested positive for an STD and could possibly infect another person through sexual activity.

MT   **Mont. Code Ann § 50-18-112 (1997)** makes it a misdemeanor for a person infected with an STD to knowingly expose another person to infection.

NY   **N.Y. Public Health Law § 2307 (McKinney 1993)** makes it a misdemeanor when any person who knowingly is infected with an STD has sexual intercourse with another person.

SC   **S.C. Code Ann. § 44-29-60 (Law. Co-op 1997)** declares that STDs are contagious, infectious, communicable and dangerous to public health. Makes it unlawful for anyone infected with STDs to knowingly expose another to infection.

TN   **Tenn. Code Ann. § 68-10-107 (1996)** prohibits any person infected with an STD to expose another person to such infection.

WA   **Wash. Rev. Code Ann. § 70.24.140 (1996)** makes it unlawful for a person who has an STD to have sex unless the partner of the infected person has been informed.

WY   **Wyo. Stat. § 35-4-132 (1997)** requires notifying an employee who is at risk of exposure to a dangerous or life-threatening STD or involved in the supervision, care and treatment of an individual infected or reasonably suspected of being infected with an STD.

Definitions

(Note: Only states that defined sexually transmitted diseases as "sexually transmitted diseases" or "venereal disease" are listed here. In addition, some specific STDs and other STD relevant terms are defined.)

CA   **Cal. Health & Safety Code § 120500 (West 1996)** defines "venereal diseases" as syphilis, gonorrhea, chancroid, lymphopathia, venereum, and granuloma inguinale.

CA   **Cal. Health & Safety Code § 120675 (West 1996)** defines "approved laboratory" as a laboratory approved by the department to conduct a syphilis test or any other laboratory where the director is licensed by the department.

CA   **Cal. Health & Safety Code § 120680 (West 1996)** defines "standard laboratory blood test" as a test for syphilis approved by the department.

DE   **Del. Code Ann. tit. 16, § 701 (1996)** defines "STD," "suspect," "director," "invasive medical procedure," "health care professional," and "healthy facility."

FL   **Fla. Stat. Ann. § 384.23 (West 1993 and Supplemental 1998)** defines "department," "county health department" and "sexually transmissible disease." Defines "STD" as a bacterial, viral, fungal or parasitic disease that is sexually transmissible and poses a threat to the public health and welfare.

HI   **Hawaii Rev. Stat. § 321-115 (1993 and Supplemental 1997)** defines "prophylactics" and outlines the guidelines for publicly vending prophylactics.

ID   **Idaho Code § 39-601 (1993)** defines "venereal diseases" as syphilis, gonorrhea, HIV/AIDS, AIDS related complexes (ARC), chancroid and Hepatitis B and are considered contagious, infectious, communicable and dangerous to public health. Makes it unlawful for anyone infected with a venereal disease to knowingly expose another person to the infection.

ID   **Idaho Code § 39-1003 (1993)** defines a "standard serological test for syphilis" as a standard serological test for syphilis by the department.

IL   **Ill. Ann. Stat. ch. 410 § 325/3 (Smith-Hurd 1997)** defines "department," "local health authority," and "sexually transmitted disease." Defines "STD" as a bacterial, viral, fungal, or parasitic disease, determined to be sexually transmissible and to be a threat to the public health and welfare.

IN   **Ind. Code Ann. § 16-41-15-2 (Burns 1993)** defines "standard serological test for syphilis" as a standard serological test for syphilis by the department.

IA   **Iowa Code § 140.2 (1997)** defines "venereal diseases" as syphilis, gonorrhea, chancroid, granuloma inguinale and lymphogranuloma venereum.

KY   **Ky. Rev. Stat. § 214.410 (1995)** defines "sexually transmitted disease" as syphilis, gonorrhea, chancroid, granuloma inguinale, genital herpes, nongonococcal urethritis, mucopurulent cervicitis, AIDS, HIV infection, chlamydia trachomatis infections and any other sexually transmitted diseases.

MI   **Mich. Stat. Ann. § 14.15 (5101) (Law. Co-op 1995)** defines a "serious communicable disease or infection" as HIV infection, AIDS, venereal disease and tuberculosis. Defines "venereal disease" as syphilis, gonorrhea, chancroid, lymphogranuloma verereum, granuloma inguinale, and other STDs that the department may rule and require to be reported.

MT   **Mont. Code Ann. § 50-19-101 (1997)** defines "STDs" as HIV, syphilis, gonorrhea, chancroid, chlamydia genital infections, lymphogranuloma verereum and granuloma inguinale. Defines STDs further as contagious, infectious, communicable and dangerous to public health.

NE   **Neb. Rev. Stat. § 71-502.01 (1996)** defines "STDs" as contagious, infectious, communicable and dangerous to the public health and includes syphilis, gonorrhea, chancroid and other STDs that the department specifies.

NJ   **N.J. Stat. Ann. § 26:4-27 (West 1996)** defines "venereal disease" as syphilis, gonorrhea, chancroid, lymphogranuloma venereum and granuloma inguinale. Defines "treating a venereal disease" and "licensed health officer."

NJ   **N.J. Stat. Ann. § 26:4-28 (West 1996)** declares syphilis, gonorrhea, chancroid, lymphogranuloma venereum and granuloma inguinale to be infectious, communicable diseases and a danger to public health.

OK   **Okla. Stat. Ann. tit. 63, § 1-236 (1997)** defines terms used in administering the state plan. Declares that the purpose of the plan is to provide a comprehensive, coordinated, multidisciplinary and interagency effort to reduce the rate of adolescent pregnancy and STDs in the state.

RI   **R.I. Gen. Laws § 23-11-1 (1996)** defines "STDs" as syphilis, gonorrhea, chancroid, granuloma inguinale and lymphogranuloma venereum and other diseases the director of health determines to constitute an STD.

SC   **S.C. Code Ann. § 44-29-60 (Law. Co-op 1997)** makes it a misdemeanor for any marriage license applicant, physician, governmental or laboratory representative to misrepresent any facts or break confidentiality about any syphilis record or lab report.

SD   **S.D. Codified Laws Ann. § 34-23-1 (1994)** defines syphilis, gonorrhea and chancroid as venereal diseases that are contagious, infectious, communicable and dangerous to public health. Makes it a Class 2 misdemeanor for anyone infected with a venereal disease to expose another person to the infection.

TN   **Tenn. Code Ann. § 68-10-112 (1996)** defines certain words used in regulating STDs. Defines an "STD" as any disease that is transmitted primarily through sexual practices and is identified in the rules and regulations of the department.

UT   **Utah Code Ann. § 26-6-16 (1995)** defines "syphilis, gonorrhea, lymphogranuloma inguinale and chancroid" as infectious diseases that are contagious, infectious, communicable and dangerous to the public health.

VT   **Vt. Stat. Ann. tit. 18, § 1091 (1982)** defines "venereal disease" as syphilis, gonorrhea and any other STD that the department determines need to be controlled.

VT   **Vt. Stat. Ann. tit. 18, § 1091a (1982)** states that venereal diseases are contagious, infectious, communicable and dangerous to public health. Requires that any person infected with a venereal disease be identified and treated for the protection of the public.

VT   **Vt. Stat. Ann. tit. 18, § 1104 (1982)** defines a "serological syphilis test" as a test approved by the board and performed by the state laboratory.

VA   **Va. Code § 32.1-55 (1997)** defines "venereal diseases" as syphilis, gonorrhea, chancroid, granuloma inguinale, lymphogranuloma venereum and any other STDs determined by the board to be dangerous to the public health.

WA   **Wash. Rev. Code Ann. § 70.24.017 (1996)** defines terms used in regulating STDs. Defines an "STD" as a bacterial, viral, fungal or parasitic disease, determined by the board by rule to be sexually transmitted and a threat to the public health and welfare.

WV   **W. Va. Code § 16-4-1 (1995)** defines syphilis, gonorrhea and chancroid as venereal diseases that are infectious, contagious, communicable and dangerous to the public health. Declares prostitution to be the prolific source of venereal diseases, and declares repression of prostitution a health measure.

Education and Prevention

AL   **Ala. Code § 16-40A-2 (1995)** requires school curriculum about sex education or human reproduction to include and emphasize abstinence from sexual intercourse as the most effective protection against unwanted pregnancy, STDs and HIV/AIDS.

AL   **Ala. Code § 22-11A-20 (1997)** requires that a physician provide information on preventing the spread of an STD when informing a person of his or her STD infection and emphasizing the necessity of treatment until cured.

CA   **Cal. Health & Safety Code § 120505 (West 1996)** requires the department to develop a program for the prevention and control of venereal diseases.

CA   **Cal. Health & Safety Code § 120510 (West 1996)** requires the department to cooperate with other institutions, facilities and agencies in preventing, controlling and curing venereal diseases.

CA   **Cal. Health & Safety Code § 120515 (West 1996)** requires the department to investigate conditions and procedures related to the prevention and control of venereal diseases. Requires the dissemination of educational information.

CA   **Cal. Health & Safety Code § 120520 (West 1996)** requires the department to conduct educational and publicity on the prevention and control of STDs.

CA   **Cal. Health & Safety Code § 120575 (West 1996)** authorizes local health officers to take all necessary measures to prevent the transmission of infection.

CA   **Cal. Health & Safety Code § 120750 (West 1996)** requires the department to develop and distribute educational information regarding venereal diseases.

CO   **Colo. Rev. Stat. § 25-4-408 (1997)** requires the department to prepare and distribute free information about the dangers of venereal diseases, how to prevent them, and the necessity for treatment. Requires any physician who examines or treats a person with a venereal disease to instruct the infected person on how to prevent the spread of the disease, the necessity for treatment and to give a free copy of information regarding venereal diseases.

FL   **Fla. Stat. Ann. § 232.246(I) (West 1989 and Supplement 1998)** requires all ninth or 10th graders be given a course in life management skills to at least include information about the prevention of HIV/AIDS and other STDs, sexual abstinence and the consequences of teenage pregnancy, drug education and the hazards of smoking.

GA   **Ga. Code Ann. § 20-2-143 (1996)** requires the state Board of Education to determine and prescribe the minimum requirements and grade level for a sex education and AIDS prevention course. Requires the state include instruction on peer pressure, promoting high self-esteem, abstinence from sexual activity as an effective method of prevention of pregnancy, STDs and AIDS. Requires each local board to authorize and develop the course on sex education and AIDS prevention. Allows a parent or legal guardian to excuse a student from sex education and AIDS prevention instruction.

GA   **Ga. Code Ann. § 26-4-7 (1982)** requires that the law does not prohibit the sale through vending machines or otherwise any articles or devices preventing venereal disease.

HI   **Hawaii Rev. Stat. § 321-111 (1993)** provides guidelines for the education and prevention of STDs through the Department of Health and the Department of Education. Requires the departments to cooperate with other public and private authorities for the education and prevention of STDs. Requires the Department of Health to coordinate an education program for preventing, detecting and encouraging early treatment of STDs. Authorizes the dissemination of STD information to minors who request it without parental consent. Authorizes the distribution of educational material to public school counselors.

IL   **Ill. Ann. Stat. ch. 105 § 5/27-9.2 (Smith-Hurd 1993)** requires a course in comprehensive sex education be offered to grades six through 12 and include instruction on the prevention and transmission and spread of AIDS. Requires all public elementary, junior high and senior high school classes that teach sex education to discuss and emphasize that abstinence from sexual intercourse is the only protection that is 100 percent effective against unwanted teenage pregnancy, STDs and HIV/AIDS. Requires providing pupils with statistics based on the latest medical information citing the failure and success rates of condoms in preventing AIDS and other STDs. Requires no student participate in any sex education that includes STDs and HIV when the parent objects. Requires any parent or guardian have the right to examine the instructional materials for sex education.

IL   Ill. Ann. Stat. ch. 105 § 5/27-9.2 (Smith-Hurd 1993) requires the state superintendent of education develop a procedure evaluating and measuring the effectiveness of sex education, including the reduction of sexual activity, STDs and premarital pregnancy among students.

IL   Ill. Ann. Stat. ch. 410 § 70/5 (Smith-Hurd 1997) requires minimum requirements for hospitals providing emergency services to sexual assault survivors. Hospitals must offer sexual assault survivors a blood test to determine the presence of an STD, written and oral instructions indicating the need for a second blood test six weeks after the sexual assault to determine the presence or absence of an STD, appropriate oral and written information about the possibility of infection of an STD and pregnancy resulting from the sexual assault, oral and written information about accepted medical procedures and medication available for the prevention or treatment of a venereal disease infection resulting from a sexual assault and information to provide or refer the victim to counseling.

IL   Ill. Ann. Stat. ch. 20 § 2310/55.55 (Smith-Hurd 1993) requires the department to distribute a brochure about STDs. Requires the brochures to be distributed free of charge to each county clerk's office and to other offices where applications for marriage licenses are taken.

IN   Ind. Code Ann. § 16-41-15-3 (Burns 1993) allows a local board or health officer to request funding for a venereal disease prevention and control program when the health officer assesses and determines that a rise of venereal disease cases that may be dangerous to the public health and safety.

IN   Ind. Code Ann. § 20-10.1-4-11 (Burns 1996) outlines the mandatory STD curriculum for elementary and secondary schools. Requires an accredited school to teach abstinence from sexual activity outside of marriage. States that abstinence is the only certain way to avoid out-of-wedlock pregnancy and STDs and that the best way to avoid STDs and other associated health problems is to have a faithful, monogamous marriage.

IN   Ind. Code Ann. § 31-11-4-5 (Burns 1997) requires the circuit court clerk to distribute information about STDs to marriage license applicants. Outlines what the information must include. Requires the circuit court clerk to state that the applicants may be tested on a voluntary basis for HIV. Allows for a religious exemption to receiving information about STDs.

LA   La. Rev. Stat. Ann § 1067 (West 1992) requires the secretary of the department to make rules and regulations for the diagnosis, treatment, reporting and prevention of venereal diseases.

LA   La. Rev. Stat. Ann § 1300.71 (West Supplemental 1998) requires the department to prepare an annual health report card indicating the overall state of health in Louisiana. Requires the report card to include state information about teenage pregnancy, birth rates, rates of low birth-weight babies, suicide rates, drug addiction, STDs and other health findings.

LA   La. Rev. Stat. Ann § 2198.2 (West Supplemental 1998) requires the rural health care authority to establish six commissions to research, develop and improve the health services for adolescents and special population groups and reduce STDs and teenage pregnancies.

MI   Mich. Stat. Ann. § 14.15 (5119) (Law. Co-op 1995) requires a marriage applicant be counseled by a physician or other authorized medical personnel on the transmission and prevention of venereal diseases and HIV infection. Requires a county clerk to distribute to each applicant educational materials prepared by the department about testing and counseling for venereal diseases and HIV. Prohibits a county clerk from issuing a marriage license to an applicant who fails to present a certificate indicating the applicant has received counseling regarding the transmission and prevention of venereal diseases and HIV from a physician and has been offered or referred for venereal disease or HIV testing.

MN   Minn. Stat. § 144.065 (1996) requires the state commissioner of health to assist local health agencies and organizations to develop services for the detection and treatment of venereal diseases. Requires these agencies to provide services for the diagnosis and treatment of venereal diseases and provide appropriate educational information. Requires the state commissioner to provide rules and technical assistance on providing services and establish a method of providing funds to these agencies.

MN   Minn. Stat. § 611A.20 (1996) requires a hospital to give written information about STDs to a person receiving medical services who reports or shows evidence of sexual assault or unwanted sexual contact. Requires the contents to inform the victim of the risk of contracting STDs as a result of a sexual assault, the symptoms of

STDs, recommendations for periodic testing for STDs, where confidential testing is done, and information necessary to make an informed decision about whether to request a test of the offender.

MS   **Miss. Code Ann. § 41-23-30 (1993)** requires the county health departments to provide free testing and treatment for STDs. Requires all testing and treatment be held confidential. Requires using available media to advertise the confidentiality of the test and treatment.

MT   **Mont. Code Ann. § 50-18-102 (1997)** authorizes the department to prevent, control and prescribe treatment for STDs and to conduct educational campaigns.

MT   **Mont. Code Ann. § 50-18-103 (1997)** requires the department to cooperate with federal agencies regarding the prevention, control and treatment of STDs. Allows the department to expend federal funds made available to the state for the prevention, control and treatment of STDs.

NE   **Neb. Rev. Stat. § 71-502.02 (1996)** requires the department to adopt rules and regulations that are necessary to control and suppress STDs.

NV   **Nev. Rev. Stat. § 441A.240 (1993)** requires the health division to control, prevent, treat and, whenever possible, ensure the cure of STDs. Requires the health division to provide materials and the curriculum necessary to conduct an educational program and to establish a program for the certification of persons qualified to instruct the program.

NV   **Nev. Rev. Stat. § 441A.250 (1993)** allows the health division to establish and provide financial assistance or other support to clinics and dispensaries for the prevention, control and treatment or cure of STDs.

NV   **Nev. Rev. Stat. § 441A.270 (1993)** requires a physician, clinic or dispensary providing treatment to a person who has an STD to teach the methods of preventing the spread of the disease and emphasize the necessity of treatment.

NH   **N.H. Rev. Stat. Ann. § 186:11 and 189:10 (1989)** requires HIV/STD education be taught in schools. Requires the state board of education to investigate the efficiency of teaching about alcohol, drugs and preventing venereal diseases and report the findings in a biennial report.

NJ   **N.J. Stat. Ann. § 26:4-34 (West 1996)** requires a physician to provide a person with a venereal disease with information about preventing the spread of the disease and the necessity for treatment. Requires the physician provide the infected person with printed instructions for preventing a venereal disease infection.

NJ   **N.J. Stat. Ann. § 26:4-47 (West 1996)** allows free diagnosis and treatment of STDs to be provided by the state department of health. Allows the commissioner of health to establish rules and regulations pertaining to the payment for services and educational materials provided by the department.

NC   **N.C. Gen. Stat. § 115C-81 (1997)** requires a comprehensive school health program be developed and administered to students in kindergarten through ninth grade that is age-appropriate, including information about preventing STDs, HIV/AIDS and other communicable diseases. Requires the state board of education to make available to all local school administrators and parents the comprehensive health education objectives, state-approved textbooks, and other state-developed or approved material that is intended to impart information or promote discussion or understanding in preventing STDs and HIV/AIDS.

OH   **Ohio Rev. Code Ann. § 3313.60 (Page 1997)** requires venereal disease education be included in the health education curriculum requirement for graduation from high school. Allows a parent or guardian to excuse the student from venereal disease instruction.

OK   **Okla. Stat. Ann. tit. 63, § 1-237 (1997)** creates the Joint Legislative Committee for Review of Coordination of Efforts for Prevention of Adolescent Pregnancy and STDs and the Interagency Coordinating Council for Coordination of Efforts for Prevention of Adolescent Pregnancy. Outlines appointment requirements for the committees, duties and objectives. Requires the joint committee to meet with state officials and employees responsible for providing services relating to the prevention of adolescent pregnancy and STDs on a regular basis, evaluate successful programs throughout the nation, recommend changes in proposed interagency agreements and the state plan, review interagency agreements and the state plan, hold hearings regarding STDs and teen pregnancy, monitor and implement the state plan, and recommend legislation to correct any upcoming problems in implementing the plan.

OK   **Okla. Stat. Ann. tit. 63, § 1-238 (1997)** creates coordination of efforts for the prevention of adolescent pregnancy and STDs. Requires the plan be a comprehensive, coordinated, multidisciplinary and an interagency effort to reduce the rate of adolescent pregnancy and STDs in the state. Requires components of the plan to a include a public awareness campaign, identification of prevention strategies and resources, coordination and collaboration among related efforts and programs, empowerment of local community prevention efforts, and evaluation of prevention strategies and programs. Requires the public awareness campaign promote abstinence from premarital sex and requires that the campaign cannot directly or indirectly condone premarital or promiscuous sexual activity.

OK   **Okla. Stat. Ann. tit. 63, § 1-526 (1997)** requires the state board of health to make rules and regulations for the control and prevention of the spread of venereal diseases.

OK   **Okla. Stat. Ann. tit. 63, § 1-528 (1997)** requires a physician who examines or treats a person with a venereal disease, to instruct the infected person on how to prevent the spread of the disease and the necessity for treatment. Requires a physician or other person who suspects that a person who has a venereal disease is exposing others to the infection to notify the local health officer.

OR   **Or. Rev. Stat. § 336.455 (1995)** requires that the integral part of health education curriculum include information about responsible sexual behaviors and hygienic practices that eliminate or reduce the risks of pregnancy, exposure of HIV, Hepatitis B and other infectious STDs. Requires the health education course teaching human sexuality or HIV in any public elementary or secondary school emphasize that abstinence from sexual contact is the only method that is 100 percent effective against unintended pregnancy, STDs and HIV.

RI   **R.I. Gen. Laws § 23-1-36.1 (1996)** requires the director of health to prepare and submit to each marriage license clerk's office in each town a packet of health information including information about STDs and an "AIDS testing and notification form." Requires that the form state that the department provides confidential free HIV tests, pre-test and post-test educational materials and post-test counseling for the HIV-positive person.

SC   **S.C. Code Ann. § 59-32-20 (Law. Co-op 1990)** requires the board to develop a comprehensive health education instructional unit that must include reproductive health education, family life education, pregnancy prevention education and STD prevention.

SC   **S.C. Code Ann. § 59-32-30 (Law. Co-op 1990)** outlines guidelines for implementing a comprehensive health education unit for students in grades K-12. Requires that for grades six through eight, the comprehensive health education unit should include information about STDs as part of the instruction. Requires that for grades nine through 12 that the program not include a discussion of an alternate sexual lifestyle except in the context of STDs.

TN   **Tenn. Code Ann. § 49-6-1008 (1996)** requires all educational materials directed toward school children that pertain to the prevention of AIDS and other STDs place primary emphasis on abstinence from premarital intimacy and avoidance of drug abuse in controlling the spread of AIDS. Requires AIDS education programs to be adopted by the local boards of education.

TN   **Tenn. Code Ann. § 68-10-103 (1996)** requires a physician or other person treating persons infected with an STD to provide information regarding STDs. Requires the information be furnished by the department.

TX   **Tex. Public Education Code Ann. § 28.004 (Vernon 1996)** requires any educational course material and instruction relating to teaching human sexuality, STDs or HIV/AIDS be selected by the local school district board of trustees. Requires all course material directed toward school children emphasize abstinence from sexual activity as the only method that is 100 percent effective in preventing pregnancy, STDs and HIV.

TX   **Tex. Health & Safety Code Ann. § 81.090 (Vernon 1992)** requires a physician to take a blood sample of a pregnant woman at the first examination and within 24 hours of the delivery and submit the sample to a certified laboratory for a standard serological test for syphilis and a standard serological test for HIV. Outlines other duties required during the first exam including distributing information about HIV/AIDS and syphilis, verbally notifying the woman that an HIV test will be performed, and advising the woman that the result of the test is not anonymous and explaining the difference between an anonymous and confidential test. Prohibits the physician from conducting the HIV test if the woman objects to the test. Requires the physician to refer the woman to an anonymous testing site or instruct the woman about anonymous testing methods, if she objects to testing.

VT   **Vt. Stat. Ann. tit. 18, § 1097 (1982)** requires the board to conduct an educational campaign on the methods used for the prevention and treatment of a person infected with a venereal disease.

VA   **Va. Code § 32.1-56 (1997)** requires a physician or any other person who examines or treats a person having a venereal disease to provide information to the infected person about the disease, the nature of the disease, methods of treatment, prevention of the spread of the disease, and the necessity of tests to ensure that a cure has been accomplished.

WA   **Wash. Rev. Code Ann. § 70.24.200 (1996)** requires that all information on STDs paid for by the state and directed toward the general public emphasize the importance of sexual abstinence, sexual fidelity and avoidance of substance abuse in controlling sexually transmitted disease.

WA   **Wash. Rev. Code Ann. § 70.24.210 (1996)** requires all material about STDs directed toward school children in grades K-12 emphasize the importance of sexual abstinence outside marriage and avoidance of substance abuse in controlling STDs.

WI   **Wis. Stat. Ann. § 115.35 (West 1991 and Supplemental 1997)** requires a "health problems education program" be integrated into the school curriculum. Requires the program to educate students about health problems which include human growth and development, controlled substances, alcohol, tobacco, STDs and HIV/AIDS.

WI   **Wis. Stat. Ann. § 252.10 (West Supplemental 1997)** requires the department to prepare information and instruction concerning STDs. Requires the information to be free upon request to state residents.

Funding

AL   **Ala. Code § 22-11A-18 (1997)** establishes a procedure for the isolation of a person infected with an STD when testing and treatment is refused. Requires the state to cover the costs of testing and treatment when an infected person is unable to pay. Allows quarantining persons who are deemed a danger to public health.

AK   **Alaska Stat. § 18.15.320** requires the cost for testing a person charged with a sex offense for HIV and other STDs be paid by the department. Requires the court to order the person to pay for the tests if convicted of the sex offense charge.

CT   **Conn. Gen. Stat. § 4-106 (1997)** Prohibits any hospital that receives state aid from refusing to admit and treat a patient suffering from a venereal disease.

CT   **Conn. Gen. Stat. § 54-102a (1997)** allows a court to order persons charged with certain sexual offenses to a venereal examination and HIV testing. Requires reporting the results to the department. Allows the court to order treatment if HIV or a venereal disease is found. Requires the examination or test be paid for by the department. Makes it a class C misdemeanor for any person who fails to comply with any court-ordered testing or treatment.

FL   **Fla. Stat. Ann. § 384.288 (West 1993 and Supplemental 1998)** outlines fees and other compensation for services required during the hospitalization, physical examination and treatment of a person infected with an STD.

HI   **Hawaii Rev. Stat. § 325-52 (1993)** outlines serologic testing and reporting. Requires requested tests to be free of charge when completed at a department laboratory. Requires the department to issue a "laboratory report form." Outlines the procedure for reporting.

IN   **Ind. Code Ann. § 16-41-15-3 (Burns 1993)** allows a local board or health officer to request funding for a venereal disease prevention and control program when the health officer assesses and determines a rise of venereal disease cases that may be dangerous to the public health and safety.

IN   **Ind. Code Ann. § 16-41-15-5 (Burns 1993 and Supplemental)** allows annual levy tax of no more than 3 cents to each $100 of taxable property to be used for the control and prevention of venereal diseases. Requires that, in 2001, the tax be lowered to 1 cent for each $100 taxable property. Requires the amount be credited to the local board's venereal disease prevention and control fund.

MA   **Mass. Gen. Laws Ann. ch. 111, § 117 (West 1996)** requires the department, along with cooperation from local boards or hospitals, establish and maintain clinics for treating venereal diseases for any person unable to pay. Allows cities and towns, through their boards, to establish clinics. Requires treatment in a clinic to include providing transportation or the reasonable cost of transportation to and from the place for the patient who is unable to pay.

MA   **Mass. Gen. Laws Ann. ch. 111, § 118** requires that no discrimination be made against a person who is receiving treatment for a venereal disease in a hospital supported by city taxes.

MS   **Miss. Code Ann. § 99-37-25 (Supplement 1997)** requires the county pay for the STD tests and medical examination of an alleged sex offender. Requires the test results be made available to the victim or to the parent or guardian of the victim if the victim is a child. Requires any defendant who is convicted of rape, sexual battery of a child, touching or handling of a child or exploiting a child pay the county for the STD tests and medical examination.

MT   **Mont. Code Ann. § 50-18-103 (1997)** requires the department to cooperate with federal agencies regarding the prevention, control and treatment of STDs. Allows the department to expend federal funds made available to the state for the prevention, control and treatment of STDs.

NV   **Nev. Rev. Stat. § 441A.250 (1993)** allows the health division to establish and provide financial assistance or other support to clinics and dispensaries for the prevention, control and treatment, or cure of STDs.

NV   **Nev. Rev. Stat. § 441A.260 (1993)** allows the health divisions to provide medical supplies and financial aid for the STD treatment of indigent patients. Requires physicians, clinics or dispensaries that accept supplies or aid to comply with all conditions prescribed by the board.

NJ   **N.J. Stat. Ann. § 26:4-46 (West 1996)** allows any person suffering from a venereal disease and who is unable to pay for treatment to apply for care and treatment. Requires the board to pay for treatment when a person is unable to pay.

NM   **N. M. Stat. Ann. § 30-9-5 (1994)** allows the court to order a venereal disease examination and treatment for a person convicted of prostitution or soliciting a prostitute. Requires the state to pay for medical treatment when the infected person is unable to pay.

PA   **Pa. Cons. Stat. Ann. tit. 35, 521.9 (Purdon 1993)** requires the department to provide free diagnosis and treatment for anyone with a venereal disease. Allows any local board or department to share in the financial support for providing free diagnosis and treatment for a venereal disease.

PR   **P.R. Laws Ann. tit. 24, § 579 (1993)** allows the department to establish STD clinics.

PR   **P.R. Laws Ann. tit. 24, § 581 (1993)** authorizes the secretary of health to accept financial assistance other than federal assistance to meet STD prevention and treatment goals of the commonwealth.

RI   **R.I. Gen. Laws § 23-11-13 (1996)** requires the General Assembly to annually appropriate money necessary for controlling the spread of STDs.

Hepatitis B

AK   **Alaska Stat. § 18.15.250** requires the department to establish a free vaccination program for Hepatitis B for all volunteer medical and rescue personnel and law enforcement officers.

CA   **Cal. Health & Safety Code § 120875 (West)** requires the department of education to provide information to school districts on AIDS, on AIDS-related conditions, and on Hepatitis B.

CA   **Cal. Health & Safety Code § 125100 (West 1996)** requires prenatal care providers and laboratories to provide the department with information necessary to evaluate the effectiveness of testing and follow-up treatment for the prevention of perinatally transmitted Hepatitis B. Mandates the department to make available, depending on funding, money to counties who request funding for testing and follow-up treatment for preventing perinatally transmitted Hepatitis B infection.

CA   **Cal. Health & Safety Code § 125105 (West 1996)** requires that Hepatitis B test results remain confidential.

ID   **Idaho Code § 39-604 (Supplemental 1997)** requires testing and treating any person imprisoned in any state correctional facility for a venereal disease and HIV. Requires testing and treating for a venereal disease of any person confined in any county or city jail when public health officials think there was exposure to an infection. Requires testing any person, including a juvenile, for HIV and Hepatitis B when charged with a sex offense or prostitution. Requires the court to release the test results to the victim or to the parent or guardian when the victim is a minor. Requires a prisoner to be entitled to HIV counseling when tested HIV positive and to receive referrals to appropriate health care and support services. Requires the victim to receive counseling and referral services at the time of the test results.

IN   **Ind. Code Ann. § 16-41-14-11 (Burns 1993)** specifies that a practitioner or other authorized person is not required to perform any tests for HIV, syphilis or Hepatitis B on a donor's semen if the semen has been previously tested as required, and evidence is submitted that the donor has been tested and all tests were negative.

IN   **Ind. Code Ann. § 16-41-14-5 (Burns 1993)** requires the practitioner to test each semen donor for syphilis, Hepatitis B and HIV before the donor provides a donation. Requires a practitioner to test each recipient initially and at least annually as long as artificial insemination procedures are continuing. Requires a practitioner to report all positive results to the department.

IN   **Ind. Code Ann. § 16-41-14-14 (Burns 1997)** requires a practitioner to keep a record of the information of semen used in artificial insemination including any HIV, syphilis or Hepatitis B test results. Allows records kept to be made available to the state department for inspection. Allows the department to enter and inspect a practitioner's facility to investigate the premises, books and records. Prohibits any person from interfering with the performance of the department.

KS   **Kan. Stat. Ann § 65-153f (Supplemental 1997)** requires a physician or a person attending a pregnant woman, with the consent of the woman, to take a blood sample for a serological test for syphilis and Hepatitis B within 14 days after the diagnosis of pregnancy. Requires an approved laboratory report all positive or reactive tests. Requires all laboratory reports, files and records to be confidential and only be opened by authorized health officers or by written consent of the woman.

MI   **Mich. Stat. Ann. § 14.15 (5111) (Law. Co-op 1995)** authorizes the department to establish reporting requirements for serious communicable diseases. Allows the department to require a licensed health professional or health facility to report a serious communicable disease or infection within 24 hours of diagnosis. Requires local health departments to furnish care for tuberculosis and venereal diseases. Requires the department to provide rules for the confidentiality of reports, records and data pertaining to the testing, care, treatment, reporting and research associated with tuberculosis, Hepatitis B and other venereal diseases.

MI   **Mich. Stat. Ann. § 14.15 (5123) (Law. Co-op 1995)** requires a physician to take blood samples of a pregnant woman and submit the specimens to an approved laboratory for HIV, Hepatitis B and venereal disease tests. Requires testing the woman at the time of delivery if the tests have not already been completed. Allows for exemption if the tests are medically inadvisable or the woman refuses to be tested.

MO   **Mo. Ann. Stat. § 210.030 (Vernon 1996)** requires a physician or a qualified medical person to take a blood sample of a pregnant woman within 20 days of her first examination and submit it to an approved laboratory for a standard serological test for syphilis and Hepatitis B. Requires the test to be free of charge.

74

MO   **Mo. Ann. Stat. § 210.040 (Vernon 1996)** requires reporting any positive syphilis or Hepatitis B tests to the department. Requires the report to be held confidential.

MO   **Mo. Ann. Stat. § 210.050 (Vernon 1996)** requires reporting on the birth or stillbirth certificate that blood tests for syphilis and Hepatitis B were made and the date of the tests. Prohibits the certificate to state the result of the tests.

MO   **Mo. Ann. Stat. § 210.060 (Vernon 1996)** makes it a misdemeanor for any licensed physician, midwife, registered nurse or other person who provides health care to a pregnant woman and who misrepresents the facts required for reporting any positive blood tests for syphilis or Hepatitis B. Requires that the crime be punishable by imprisonment of no more than a year, or by a fine of no more than $1,000, or both.

NC   **N.C. Gen. Stat. § 15A-615 (1997)** allows testing a sex offender who has had an alleged sexual contact with any minor under 16 years of age for STDs, including chlamydia, gonorrhea, Hepatitis B, herpes, HIV and syphilis. Allows the victim to petition the court for the offender to be tested. Requires the test results be reported to the local health director. Requires the victim and alleged offender be informed of the tests results and be provided with counseling. Requires the results of the test not be admissible as evidence in any criminal proceeding.

SC   **S.C. Code Ann. § 16-15-255 (Law. Co-op 1997)** requires testing of certain sex offenders for Hepatitis B, STDs and HIV. Outlines court procedures. Requires the convicted offender to pay for the test unless the offender is indigent, then the tests will be paid for by the state. Requires the state provide the victim and the convicted offender with counseling if any of the tests are positive.

SC   **S.C. Code Ann. § 16-3-740 (Law. Co-op 1997)** requires testing of certain convicted offenders for Hepatitis B, STDs and HIV within 15 days of the conviction. Outlines court procedures. Requires the convicted offender or adjudicated juvenile offender to pay for the test unless the offender is indigent, then the tests will be paid for by the state. Requires the state to provide the victim and the convicted offender with counseling if any of the tests are positive.

TN   **Tenn. Code Ann. § 68-10-116 (1996)** allows an officer to request an arrested person's blood be tested for the presence of Hepatitis B or HIV if the officer is exposed during the arresting, transporting or processing of a person. Requires testing to occur at a licensed health care facility, with the cost to be paid by the division that employs the law enforcement officer. Requires the test be confidential and allows the officer exposed to request the test results.

Investigation

AL   **Ala. Code § 22-11A-13 (1997)** authorizes and directs the Board of Health to declare rules for testing, reporting, investigation and treatment of STDs.

CA   **Cal. Health & Safety Code § 120565 (West 1996)** allows an agency to investigate whether a person who has discontinued treatment, has initiated or is participating in treatment elsewhere.

DE   **Del. Code Ann. tit. 16, § 703 (1996)** authorizes the director to isolate, examine, investigate and treat any person suspected of being infected with STDs. Authorizes the director to require a person infected with an STD to find treatment.

FL   **Fla. Stat. Ann. § 384.33 (West 1993)** allows the department to adopt rules regarding the investigation, treatment and confidentiality of STDs.

ID   **Idaho Code § 39-603 (1993)** authorizes any state, county and municipal health officer to investigate and examine any person reasonably suspected of being infected with a venereal disease and requires that person to report for quarantine and treatment. Requires all local and state health officers to cooperate with proper officials who enforce prostitution laws to control venereal diseases.

IL   **Ill. Ann. Stat. ch. 410 § 325/5 (Smith-Hurd 1997)** requires the department to adopt rules regarding the authorization of interviews for investigating persons infected or believed to be infected with an STD, and to order a person to submit to an examination and treatment. Requires all information gathered during an investigation be confidential. Makes it a Class A misdemeanor for any person who knowingly discloses any information of any person infected with an STD.

IL   **Ill. Ann. Stat. ch. 410 § 325/10 (Smith-Hurd 1997)** requires the department to adopt the rules necessary in performing the duties of the department. Requires rules of the department to include criteria, standards and procedures for the identification, investigation, examination and treatment of STDs.

IN   **Ind. Code Ann. § 16-41-14-14 (Burns 1997)** requires a practitioner to keep a record of the information of semen used in artificial insemination including any HIV, syphilis or Hepatitis B test results. Allows records kept to be made available to the state department for inspection. Allows the department to enter and inspect a practitioner's facility to investigate the premises, books and records. Prohibits any person from interfering with the performance of the department.

IN   **Ind. Code Ann. § 16-41-14-20 (Burns 1993)** makes it a Class B misdemeanor for a person who recklessly fails to comply or interferes with the inspection or investigation of an STD case. Constitutes a separate offense for each day a violation continues.

IA   **Iowa Code § 140.7 (1997)** authorizes the department to use every available means to investigate and determine the source and spread of any reported infectious disease case.

MT   **Mont. Code Ann. § 50-18-107 (1997)** outlines powers and duties of health officers. Authorizes health officers to examine, isolate, or investigate a person suspected of being infected with an STD. Allows only a local or state health officer to terminate a quarantine.

NE   **Neb. Rev. Stat. § 71-504 (1996)** allows a minor to obtain an examination and treatment for STDs without the consent or notification of a parent or guardian. Releases the physician from incurring any liability. Requires the parent to be held liable for treatment expenses of a minor. Authorizes interviewing an infected person to find out the names of sexual contacts so that an appropriate investigation can be made to locate and eliminate other sources of infection.

NE   **Neb. Rev. Stat. § 71-506 (1996)** makes it a Class V misdemeanor for any person who violates any STD rule or regulation of the department. Makes it a Class III misdemeanor for any person who willfully or maliciously breaks confidentiality and discloses the contents of any report, notification or investigation of an STD.

NV   **Nev. Rev. Stat. § 441A.220 (1997)** requires all information regarding the report of an STD case or the investigation of a case by the health authority be confidential and not disclosed to any person, including information used for court proceedings with exceptions. Provides exceptions.

NJ   **N.J. Stat. Ann. § 26:4-33 (West 1996)** authorizes the local board to investigate any suspected venereal disease case to identify a possible source of infection.

ND   **N.D. Cent. Code § 23-07-07 (1991)** authorizes the state, local and city health officers when necessary for the protection of public health to examine any person suspected of being infected with an STD, to require any person to report for treatment, to investigate any cases and cooperate with other officials to enforce the laws.

OK   **Okla. Stat. Ann. tit. 63, § 1-529 (1997)** authorizes the local health officers to use any means necessary to investigate and examine an infected person who has been reported two or more times as a suspected source of venereal infection.

PR   **P.R. Laws Ann. tit. 24, § 578 (1993)** requires providers to counsel, interview, and investigate anyone suspected of having an STD infection.

RI   **R.I. Gen. Laws § 23-11-10 (1996)** authorizes the department to take appropriate measures to investigate sources of STD infections. Allows full powers for the inspection, examination and treatment of all suspected STD cases and sources.

SD   **S.D. Codified Laws Ann. § 34-23-3 (1994)** requires all local and state health officers to investigate sources of venereal disease infection and to cooperate with the offices that enforce the laws against prostitution.

TN   **Tenn. Code Ann. § 68-10-104 (1996)** authorizes state, district, county and municipal health officers to investigate and examine any person reasonably suspected of being infected with an STD and requires such person to report for treatment and quarantine. Allows any state, district, county or municipal health officer, or any physician to examine, diagnose and treat minors infected with an STD without the knowledge or consent of the parents. Releases the physician or health officer from any liability except for negligence.

WA   **Wash. Rev. Code Ann. § 70.24.024 (1996)** authorizes state and local health officers or other authorized persons to examine any person believed to be infected or exposed to an STD. States restrictive measures be used as a last resort when investigating an STD case. Authorizes a health officer to order a person to submit to a medical examination, testing, counseling or treatment within 14 days of the initial investigation. Authorizes a health officer to restrict a person from any behavior or conduct that endangers the public. Requires these restrictions be in writing. Outlines issuance of the restriction order and court proceedings. Requires all information be confidential unless a public hearing is requested.

WV   **W. Va. Code § 16-4-2 (1995)** authorizes municipal and county health officers to use every available means to investigate all cases of syphilis, gonorrhea and chancroid. Allows health officers to designate any member of the police or health department to make investigations.

WV   **W. Va. Code § 16-4-9 (1995)** requires a physician or other person who examines or treats a person with syphilis, gonorrhea or chancroid to inform that person of the necessity of taking treatment and continuing the treatment as prescribed. Requires a physician to report a patient who has stopped treatment to the local health officer. Makes it a misdemeanor for anyone to stop treatment for a venereal disease. Requires the local health officer to investigate any unfinished treatments for a venereal disease. Authorizes the local health officer to arrest, detain and quarantine any patient who fails to return for treatment.

WV   **W. Va. Code § 16-4-11 (1995)** requires a physician to report and to notify the local health officer of any person who is suspected of having syphilis, gonorrhea or chancroid and is exposing others to the infection. Requires the local health officer to investigate any suspected venereal disease cases.

WV   **W. Va. Code § 16-4-12 (1995)** allows a local health officer to investigate, arrest, detain and quarantine any person who is suffering from a venereal disease in an infectious stage and is not under treatment.

WI   **Wis. Stat. Ann. § 252.10 (West Supplemental 1997)** authorizes the health authority to investigate any suspected or reported cases of STDs.

Minors—Consent to Testing and Treatment

AL   **Ala. Code § 22-8-6 (1997)** allows a minor to give consent for any medical or mental health services to determine or treat pregnancy, venereal disease, drug dependency or alcoholism.

AL   **Ala. Code § 22-11A-19 (1997)** allows minors age 12 and older to consent to medical treatment for STDs. Allows a medical provider to inform a parent or guardian about STD treatment.

AZ   **Ariz. Rev. Stat. Ann. § 44-132.01 (1994)** allows a minor to give consent for hospital or medical care for the diagnosis and treatment of a venereal disease.

AR   **Ark. Stat. Ann. § 20-16-508 (1991)** allows a minor to give consent for the examination and treatment of a venereal disease. Requires the consent of a spouse, parent or guardian not be necessary for authorizing hospital care or services provided by a licensed physician. Allows the physician to inform or give information about the treatment to the parent or guardian.

CA   **Cal. Family Code App. § 34.7 (West 1994)** allows minors age 12 and older to consent to diagnosis or medical treatment for STDs. Requires that a parent or legal guardian not be held liable for the payment of care.

CT   **Conn. Gen. Stat. § 19a-216 (1997)** allows any municipal health department, state institution or facility, licensed physician, or any public or private hospital or clinic to examine and treat a minor for a venereal disease. Requires the records of an examination and treatment of the minor be confidential and not be divulged by the facility or physician, including prohibiting sending the bill for services to any person other than the minor. Requires the minor be responsible for all costs and expenses for services. Requires reporting any venereal disease treatment of a minor younger than 12 to the commissioner of children and families.

DE   **Del. Code Ann. tit. 16, § 710 (1996)** outlines the protocol for treatment, consent and liability for payment in the care of minors for STDs. Requires records be confidential.

FL   **Fla. Stat. Ann. § 384.30 (West 1998)** outlines the protocol for the treatment and consent in the care of minors for STDs. Requires that consultation, examination and treatment of a minor for an STD remain confidential.

GA   **Ga. Code Ann. § 31-17-7 (1996)** allows a minor to consent to medical or surgical care or services for a venereal disease. Allows the physician treating the minor to inform the spouse, parent or guardian without the consent of the minor and even over the express refusal of the minor.

HI   **Hawaii Rev. Stat. § 321-111 (1993)** provides guidelines for the education and prevention of STDs through the Department of Health and the Department of Education. Requires the departments to cooperate with other public and private authorities for the education and prevention of STDs. Requires the Department of Health to coordinate an education program for preventing, detecting and encouraging early treatment of STDs. Authorizes the dissemination of STD information to minors who request it without parental consent. Authorizes the distribution of educational material to public school counselors.

HI   **Hawaii Rev. Stat. § 577A-2 (1993)** allows a minor to consent to treatment for a pregnancy, venereal disease or other medical services and requires that no other person's consent, including a spouse, parent or guardian, be necessary to authorize hospital, clinic or medical care.

HI   **Hawaii Rev. Stat. § 577A-3 (1993)** allows the physician treating a minor for a venereal disease to disclose information to the spouse, parent or guardian after consulting with the minor first about the disclosure. Allows information to be disclosed when the minor is not pregnant or infected with a venereal disease.

ID   **Idaho Code § 39-3801 (1993)** allows a minor age 14 or older to consent to hospital, medical or surgical care related to the diagnosis or treatment of a venereal disease. Requires the parent of the minor not be liable for any payment for any venereal disease care.

IL   **Ill. Ann. Stat. ch. 410 § 210/4 (Smith-Hurd 1997)** outlines the protocol for the treatment and care of minors for STDs, alcoholism and addiction. Allows a minor age 12 or older to give consent to medical care or counseling for STDs. Specifies that the consent of a parent or legal guardian is not necessary when diagnosing or treating STDs for a minor patient.

78

IL   **Ill. Ann. Stat. ch. 410 § 210/5 (Smith-Hurd 1997)** releases any physician, psychologist, social worker or other qualified person who provides diagnosis, treatment or counseling to a minor for an STD, from the obligation to inform the parent or guardian, without the minor's consent unless the action is necessary to protect the safety of the minor, family member or individual.

IA   **Iowa Code § 140.9 (1997)** allows a minor to seek diagnosis or treatment for a venereal disease without the consent of a parent. Requires medical diagnosis and treatment for the minor be given by a licensed physician.

KS   **Kan. Stat. Ann § 65-2892 (1992)** allows a minor under age 18 to consent to an examination and medical treatment for a venereal disease. Allows, but does not obligate, the physician to inform the spouse, parent or guardian of the minor being treated. Releases the physician from incurring civil or criminal liability for making an examination or treatment, except in the case of negligence.

KY   **Ky. Rev. Stat. § 214.185 (1995)** allows a minor to consent to an examination and treatment for a venereal disease, pregnancy, alcohol or drug abuse. Requires the physician to incur no civil or criminal liability, not including negligence, for examining or treating a minor. Requires a parent or guardian of the minor receiving treatment for a venereal disease not be financially responsible for the care.

LA   **La. Rev. Stat. Ann § 1065.1 (West 1992)** allows a minor to consent for treatment for a venereal disease. Allows, but does not obligate, the treating physician to inform the spouse, parent or guardian of the minor being treated for a venereal disease. Releases the physician from incurring civil or criminal liability with examination, diagnosis and treatment except in the case of negligence.

ME   **Me. Rev. Stat. Ann. tit. 22, § 1823 (1992)** allows any hospital, alcohol or drug treatment facility to provide treatment to a minor for a venereal disease without obtaining consent of the minor's parent or guardian or informing the parent or guardian. Requires the hospital to notify and obtain the consent of the minor's parent or guardian when hospitalization continues for more than 16 hours.

ME   **Me. Rev. Stat. Ann. tit. 32, § 2595 (1997)** allows an individual licensed to provide medical care to provide treatment for a venereal disease to a minor without obtaining the consent of the minor's parent or guardian. Allows the individual providing the medical care to inform the parent or guardian of the treatment.

MD   **Md. Health Code Ann. § 20-102 (1996)** allows a minor to consent to medical treatment for drug abuse, alcoholism, venereal disease, pregnancy or injuries from an alleged rape or sexual offense. Requires a physician who treats a minor not be liable for any civil or criminal activity. Allows a physician who provided treatment, care or advice to a minor for STDs to inform a spouse, parent or guardian.

MA   **Mass. Gen. Laws Ann. ch. 111, § 117 (West 1996)** requires the department, along with cooperation from local boards or hospitals, to establish and maintain clinics for treating venereal diseases for any person unable to pay. Allows cities and towns, through their boards, to establish clinics. Requires treatment in a clinic to include providing transportation or the reasonable cost of transportation to and from the place for the patient who is unable to pay.

MI   **Mich. Stat. Ann. § 14.15 (5127) (Law. Co-op 1995)** allows a minor to consent to treatment for a venereal disease or HIV. Allows a physician to inform the spouse, parent or guardian of the treatment. Requires that a spouse, parent or guardian not be financially responsible for the minor's treatment.

MN   **Minn. Stat. § 144.343 (1996)** allows a minor to consent to treatment for pregnancy, venereal disease or alcohol and drug abuse.

MS   **Miss. Code Ann. § 41-41-13 (Supplemental 1997)** allows any physician to treat a minor for a venereal disease without first obtaining the consent of or informing the parent or guardian of the treatment.

MT   **Mont. Code Ann. § 41-1-402 (1997)** allows a minor to consent to prevention, diagnosis and treatment from a licensed physician for a pregnancy, drug abuse or a venereal disease. Requires the physician treating a minor for a venereal disease to refer the minor to counseling.

MT   **Mont. Code Ann. § 41-1-403 (1997)** allows, but does not obligate, the physician to inform the spouse, parent or guardian of a minor receiving treatment for a venereal disease when severe complications are present or anticipated, major surgery or hospitalization is needed, the hospital desires a third-party commitment to pay for services, failure to inform the parent would jeopardize the safety of the minor or to inform them would benefit the minor's physical mental health. Prohibits information from being disclosed to the parent or guardian without the consent of the minor when the minor is found not to be pregnant, suffering from drug abuse or infected with an STD.

MT   **Mont. Code Ann. § 50-19-107 (1997)** requires laboratory results of an STD test be shown by the physician to the patient. Allows the report of the results to be shown, upon request of the patient, to the spouse of the patient or, if the patient is a minor, to the minor's parents or the minor's legal guardian.

NE   **Neb. Rev. Stat. § 71-504 (1996)** allows a minor to obtain an examination and treatment for STDs without the consent or notification of a parent or guardian. Releases the physician from incurring any liability. Requires the parent to be held liable for treatment expenses of a minor. Authorizes interviewing an infected person to find out the names of his or her sexual partners so that an appropriate investigation can be made to locate and eliminate other sources of infection.

NV   **Nev. Rev. Stat. § 129.60 (1993)** authorizes any local or state health officer, licensed physician or clinic to examine and treat any minor who is suspected of being infected or is found to be infected with any STD (without the consent of the parent or legal guardian).

NH   **N.H. Rev. Stat. Ann. § 141-C:18 (1996)** allows any minor 14 years of age or older to voluntarily submit to a medical diagnosis and treatment for an STD. Allows a licensed physician to diagnose, treat or prescribe medication for the treatment of an STD without the knowledge or consent of the parent or legal guardian.

NM   **N. M. Stat. Ann. § 24-1-9 (1997)** allows any person, regardless of age, to consent to an examination and treatment by a licensed physician for an STD.

NM   **N. M. Stat. Ann. § 24-1-9.1 (1997)** allows for STD testing of persons convicted of certain criminal offenses. Allows the victim of a criminal sexual offense to petition the court to order a test be performed on the offender when consent to perform a test cannot be obtained. Allows the parent or legal guardian to petition the court when the victim is a minor. Requires the court order to state that the test be administered to the offender within 10 days after the petition is filed. Requires the test results be disclosed only to the offender and the victim or the victim's parent or legal guardian.

NY   **N.Y. Public Health Law § 2305 (McKinney 1993)** prohibits any person other than a licensed physician from diagnosing, treating or prescribing medicine to a person infected with an STD. Allows a licensed physician to diagnose, treat or prescribe for a person under age 21 without the consent or knowledge of a parent or guardian.

NC   **N.C. Gen. Stat. § 90-21.5 (1997)** allows a minor to consent to the prevention, diagnosis and treatment of a venereal disease, alcohol or drug abuse or emotional disturbance from a licensed physician.

ND   **N.D. Cent. Code § 14-10-17 (1997)** allows any person age 14 or older to receive an examination and treatment for STDs, alcoholism and/or drug abuse without permission or consent of a parent or guardian.

OH   **Ohio Rev. Code Ann. § 3709. 24.1 (Page 1997)** allows a minor to give consent for the diagnosis or treatment of any venereal disease by a licensed physician. Requires parent or guardian of the minor giving consent not be held liable for payment for any diagnostic or treatment services.

OK   **Okla. Stat. Ann. tit. 63, § 1-532.1 (1997)** allows any minor, regardless of age, to consent to an examination and treatment for a venereal disease by a licensed physician.

OR   **Or. Rev. Stat. § 109.610 (1995)** allows a minor to give consent for the diagnosis or treatment of any venereal disease. Requires parent or legal guardian of the minor not be liable for payment of any medical care.

PA   **Pa. Cons. Stat. Ann. tit. 35, § 521.14a (Purdon 1993)** allows any person under age 21 who is infected with an STD to be treated by a physician. States that, if the minor consents to undergo treatment, then approval or consent of the parents is not necessary. Requires the physician not be held liable or sued for treatment of a minor.

PA   **Pa. Cons. Stat. Ann. tit. 35, § 10103 (Purdon 1993)** allows a minor to give consent for medical and health services for pregnancy or venereal disease.

RI   **R.I. Gen. Laws § 23-11-11 (1996)** authorizes the department to examine any person reasonably suspected of having an STD. Requires the department to inform the infected person of the right to have his or her own physician present. Allows any person under age 18 to give consent for the examination and treatment of an STD. Releases the physician examining the minor from any liability.

SD   **S.D. Codified Laws Ann. § 34-23-16 (1994)** allows a minor to consent to the diagnosis and treatment for a venereal disease by a licensed physician.

SD **S.D. Codified Laws Ann. § 34-23-17 (1994)** allows a county or state health department or a doctor associated with the department to treat a minor for a venereal disease without the consent or notification of the parents.

SD **S.D. Codified Laws Ann. § 34-23-18 (1994)** requires that any hospital, public clinic or licensed physician who provides the diagnosis, care or treatment of a venereal disease to a minor not incur any civil or criminal liability. Requires that immunity not apply to any negligent acts or omissions.

TN **Tenn. Code Ann. § 68-10-104 (1996)** authorizes state, district, county and municipal health officers to investigate and examine any person reasonably suspected of being infected with an STD and requires such person to report for treatment and quarantine. Allows any state, district, county, or municipal health officer or any physician to examine, diagnose and treat minors infected with an STD without the knowledge or consent of the parents. Releases the physician or health officer from any liability except for negligence.

TX **Tex. Family Code Ann § 54.033 (Vernon 1996)** outlines juvenile justice proceedings for STD and HIV testing. Requires a juvenile found delinquent of certain crimes to undergo an STD and HIV/AIDS test at the direction of the court or at the request of the victim. Allows the court to order a test if the child refuses to consent to the procedure or test. Prohibits the court from releasing the test result to anyone other than an authorized person.

UT **Utah Code Ann. § 26-6-18 (1995)** allows a minor to consent to treatment for an STD by a licensed physician or medical care provided by a hospital or public clinic.

VT **Vt. Stat. Ann. tit. 18, § 4226 (1982)** allows a minor who is at least 12 years old to consent to medical treatment and hospitalization for a venereal disease. Requires a physician to notify a parent or legal guardian if immediate hospitalization is needed for treating a venereal disease.

WA **Wash. Rev. Code Ann. § 70.24.110 (1996)** allows for a minor age 14 and older who has come in contact with any STD to give consent to diagnosis or treatment. Removes the requirement for consent of the parent or guardian and states that the parent or guardian not be held liable for payment.

WV **W. Va. Code § 16-4-10 (1995)** allows any licensed physician to examine, diagnose and treat a minor with his or her consent for any venereal disease without the knowledge or consent of the minor's parent or guardian. Requires the physician not incur any civil or criminal liability for examining, diagnosing or treating the minor.

WI **Wis. Stat. Ann. § 252.10 (West Supplemental 1997)** allows a physician to examine, diagnose and treat a minor infected with an STD without obtaining the consent of the minor's parents or guardian. States that the physician incur no liability.

WY **Wyo. Stat. § 35-4-131 (1997)** allows a person under age 18 to give legal consent for the examination and treatment of any STD infection. Requires a physician, health officer or other person, or facility providing health care to administer treatment or refer appropriate treatment of any person reasonably suspected of being infected or exposed to an STD. States that a physical examination and treatment of a consenting person under age 18 by a licensed physician or other qualified health care provider is not an assault on that person.

Miscellaneous

CA   **Cal. Health & Safety Code § 120525 (West 1996)** allows the department to establish, maintain and subsidize clinics, dispensaries and prophylactic stations for the diagnosis, treatment and prevention of venereal diseases. Requires approval of a clinic, dispensary or prophylactic station by the Board of Health.

IL   **Ill. Ann. Stat. ch. 410 § 650/10 (Smith-Hurd 1997)** prohibits any employer from requiring, allowing or permitting any person who is infected with an STD to work in a building, room or vehicle used for the production, preparation, manufacture, storage, sale or distribution of food.

MN   **Minn. Stat. § 62Q.14 (1996)** prohibits any health insurance plan from restricting the choice of an enrollee as to where the enrollee receives services related to testing and treatment of STDs.

NV   **Nev. Rev. Stat. § 441A.260 (1993)** allows the health divisions to provide medical supplies and financial aid for the STD treatment of indigent patients. Requires physicians, clinics or dispensaries that accept supplies or aid to comply with all conditions prescribed by the board.

NJ   **N.J. Stat. Ann. § 26:4-42 (West 1996)** prohibits any person with a venereal disease from nursing the sick, caring for children, or working with preparing or manufacturing milk.

NJ   **N.J. Stat. Ann. § 26:4-49.6 (West 1996)** requires a migrant laborer to submit to a syphilis, gonorrhea and venereal disease examination within 30 days after entering New Jersey to work, unless the migrant laborer can prove that a venereal disease examination was completed within the last 90 days. Requires any person who employs a migrant laborer to notify the state department of health within five days of the beginning of employment whether the person has been examined for a venereal disease.

OR   **Or. Rev. Stat. § 677.370 (1995)** prohibits any person with a venereal disease from donating sperm for the use of artificial insemination.

UT   **Utah Code Ann. § 30-1-2.3 (1997)** validates all marriages between persons who are infected with HIV/AIDS, syphilis, and/or gonorrhea prior to October 21, 1993.

WV   **W. Va. Code § 16-4-18 (1995)** makes it unlawful for any person having a venereal disease in an infectious stage to work at a barbershop, bakery, hotel or restaurant. Requires the physician reporting the venereal disease case to notify the local health officer about the employee. Makes it a misdemeanor for anyone who is infected with a venereal disease who does not stop working within 24 hours.

Notification

CA   **Cal. Health & Safety Code § 120555 (West 1996)** requires an STD-infected person to report the names and addresses of those from whom the disease may have been contracted and those who may have been infected.

CA   **Cal. Health & Safety Code § 120600-05 (West 1996)** makes it a misdemeanor for any person who refuses to give information or fails to comply with any proper control measure or examination for STDs, exposes or infects another person with an STD, or who is infected with a venereal disease who is infectious, and knows they are infected, to marry or have sexual intercourse. Specifies religious exemptions.

FL   **Fla. Stat. Ann. § 796.08 (West 1998)** requires a person already convicted of prostitution to be tested for HIV and STDs when arrested for prostitution. States the penalties for prostituting or soliciting another for prostitution while knowing of the infection and not informing the other person involved.

GA   **Ga. Code Ann. § 31-17-7 (1996)** allows a minor to consent to medical or surgical care or services for a venereal disease. Allows the physician treating the minor to inform the spouse, parent or guardian without the consent of the minor and even over the express refusal of the minor.

GA   **Ga. Code Ann. § 42-1-7 (1997)** requires any state or county correctional institution, municipal or county detention facility to notify the law enforcement agency of the transporting of an inmate or patient infected with any venereal disease, HIV or other infectious, communicable disease. Requires information released for the transporting be kept confidential and only be released or obtained by the institution, facilities or agencies that are involved with the transporting of the infected patient or inmate. Makes it a misdemeanor for any person to make any unauthorized disclosure of the transporting information.

IN   **Ind. Code Ann. § 16-41-14-9 (Burns 1993)** requires a practitioner to report the name and address of a semen donor or recipient to the department if an STD or HIV is present. Requires a practitioner to attempt to notify a donor or recipient if the semen tested is positive for STD or HIV. Requires reporting of the test results.

LA   **La. Rev. Stat. Ann § 15:535 (West 1992 and Supplemental)** authorizes the court to order an adjudicated delinquent or a person convicted of a sexual offense to submit to an STD or HIV test. Requires the procedure or test to be performed by a qualified physician who is required to report any positive result to the Department of Public Safety and Corrections. Requires notification of the test results to the victim or the parents regardless of the results.

MT   **Mont. Code Ann. § 50-18-106 (1997)** requires any physician or other person who knows or has reason to suspect that a person has an STD and might expose someone else to notify the local health officer of the name and address of the infected person.

NE   **Neb. Rev. Stat. § 71-504 (1996)** allows a minor to obtain an examination and treatment for STDs without the consent or notification of a parent or guardian. Releases the physician from incurring any liability. Requires the parent to be held liable for treatment expenses of a minor. Authorizes interviewing an infected person to find out the names of his or her sexual partners so that an appropriate investigation can be made to locate and eliminate other sources of infection.

NE   **Neb. Rev. Stat. § 71-506 (1996)** makes it a Class V misdemeanor for any person who violates any STD rule or regulation of the department. Makes it a Class III misdemeanor for any person who willfully or maliciously breaks confidentiality and discloses the contents of any report, notification or investigation of an STD.

NV   **Nev. Rev. Stat. § 441A.290 (1993)** requires a person who has an STD, if requested, to inform the health authority of the source or possible source of the infection.

NJ   **N.J. Stat. Ann. § 26:4-49.8 (West 1996)** requires examining and treating a prisoner for a venereal disease. Allows a prisoner to be isolated when a prisoner refuses treatment for a venereal disease. Requires the warden to notify the department when a prisoner with a venereal disease will be released. Requires the notification to be five days prior to the actual date of release or no later than the day following the release date.

NM   **N. M. Stat. Ann. § 24-1-8 (1997)** requires any physician who knows or has good reason to suspect that a person having an STD may expose another person to infection to notify the district health officer of the name and address of the diseased person and the facts of the case.

NM N. M. Stat. Ann. § 24-1-9.6 (1997) allows a victim of an alleged criminal offense who receives information about an STD test result to disclose the test results to protect the victim's health and safety, or the health and safety of the victim's family or sexual partner.

OK Okla. Stat. Ann. tit. 63, § 1-523 (1997) requires all correctional facilities, public or private, to have records showing all STD- and HIV-infected inmates and to keep these records on hand for one year. Requires all institutions to furnish a physician with medicine to properly treat an infected person. Requires that facilities provide all correctional employees, probation and parole officers who will have direct contact with inmates, with names of any HIV-infected inmates.

OK Okla. Stat. Ann. tit. 63, § 1-528 (1997) requires a physician who examines or treats a person with a venereal disease, to instruct the infected person on how to prevent the spread of the disease and the necessity for treatment. Requires a physician or other person who suspects a person who has a venereal disease is exposing others to the infection to notify the local health officer.

SC S.C. Code Ann. § 44-29-90 (Law. Co-op 1997) authorizes state, district, county and municipal health officers to examine, isolate and treat any person infected or suspected of being infected with an STD. Requires an infected person to report for treatment at public expense. Requires the infected person to identify anyone with whom he or she has had sexual contact, intravenous drug use, or both. Makes available state resources to be used when a person is identified as being infected with HIV/AIDS and has known sexual contacts, intravenous drug use contacts, or both. Requires notifying anyone who may have been infected and also requires the identity of the person who infected them not be revealed.

TN Tenn. Code Ann. § 68-10-102 (1996) requires physicians to notify a health officer of the name and address of an STD-infected person who is exposing others to infection.

TN Tenn. Code Ann. § 68-10-107 (1996) prohibits any person infected with an STD to expose another person to such infection.

WA Wash. Rev. Code Ann. § 70.24.022 (1996) requires the board to adopt rules authorizing interviews of all persons infected with an STD, to investigate the source, and to order an infected or believed to be infected person to submit to an examination, counseling and treatment. Requires all information gathered to be confidential. Allows a person who is reasonably believed to be infected with an STD to reveal the name or names of sexual contacts and not be held liable. Makes it a gross misdemeanor for any person who knowingly gives any false information concerning the existence of any STD.

WA Wash. Rev. Code Ann. § 70.24.105 (Supplemental 1997) prohibits any person to disclose or be compelled to disclose the identity of any person who has investigated, considered or requested a test or treatment for an STD. Allows for the exchange of medical information with certain authorized medical and social services personnel, law enforcement officers or by court order. Allows disclosure of test results upon the request of a victim of a sex crime.

WY Wyo. Stat. § 7-1-109 (1977) requires testing for STDs in sexual offense cases. Outlines court procedures. Requires examination results to be reported to the appropriate health officer. Requires the health officer to notify the victim, alleged victim or, if a minor, the parents or guardian of the victim or the alleged victim. Requires costs of any medical examination be funded through the department. Requires all results be held confidential and are inadmissible as evidence in court and will remain undisclosed except under certain circumstances.

WY Wyo. Stat. § 35-4-132 (1997) requires notifying an employee who is at risk of exposure to a dangerous or life-threatening STD or involved in the supervision, care and treatment of an individual infected or reasonably suspected of being infected with an STD.

WY Wyo. Stat. § 35-4-133 (1997) authorizes a health officer to isolate and examine an STD-infected or suspected to be an infected individual. Requires the individual to submit to treatment at public expense. Allows providing STD education information and counseling for the STD-infected individual. Requires the health officer to investigate sources of STDs and cooperate with the proper law enforcement in enforcing the laws against prostitution.

Quarantining/Isolation/Compulsory Testing and Treatment

AL   **Ala. Code § 22-11A-18 (1997)** establishes a procedure for the isolation of a person infected with an STD when testing and treatment is refused. Requires the state to cover the costs of testing and treatment when an infected person is unable to pay. Allows quarantining persons who are deemed a danger to public health.

AL   **Ala. Code § 22-11A-24 (1997)** allows a state or county health officer to petition a probate judge of the county to commit a person to the custody of the department for compulsory testing, treatment or quarantine, when any person who is exposed to an STD or where reasonable evidence indicates exposure to an STD, refuses testing or treatment, or whose conduct indicates exposure to others.

CA   **Cal. Health & Safety Code § 120570 (West 1996)** requires an agency to report to the department the name of a person who refuses to comply with treatment.

CA   **Cal. Health & Safety Code § 120585 (West 1996)** allows health officers to inspect and quarantine any place or person when found necessary to enforce the regulations of the department as they relate to STDs.

CA   **Cal. Health & Safety Code § 120595 (West 1996)** requires any physician, health officer, spouse or other person to testify in the prosecution of the violation of any rule, regulation or quarantine of an STD.

CO   **Colo. Rev. Stat. § 25-4-405 (1997)** requires any person confined, detained or imprisoned in any state or county hospital for the insane, mental institution, home for dependent children, reformatory, prison, or any private or charitable institution to be examined and treated for a venereal disease. Requires a manager to make room available to the health authorities for quarantining and treating the confined person for a venereal disease. Requires any person infected with a venereal disease at the time of their release to be quarantined and treated at public expense. Authorizes the department to arrange for hospitalization.

CO   **Colo. Rev. Stat. § 25-4-406 (1997)** requires the department to make rules and regulations providing for the quarantine, treatment and control of venereal diseases. Requires all department rules and regulations regarding venereal diseases to have the effect of law.

CT   **Conn. Gen. Stat. § 18-94 (1997)** allows keeping a prison inmate who is infected with a venereal disease in the correctional or charitable institution longer than the date of the prisoner's discharge when the institution considers the inmate to be dangerous to the public health.

DE   **Del. Code Ann. tit. 16, § 703 (1996)** authorizes the director to isolate, examine, investigate and treat any person suspected of being infected with STDs. Authorizes the director to require a person infected with an STD to find treatment.

DE   **Del. Code Ann. tit. 16, § 704 (1996)** establishes the procedure for the apprehension, commitment, treatment, quarantine and possible court hearings of an STD-infected person. Sets guidelines for anyone who refuses to comply. Allows the director of the Division of Public Health to petition the courts for an order to quarantine and treat an infected person. Outlines the procedures.

DE   **Del. Code Ann. tit. 16, § 706 (1996)** establishes protocol for the examination and treatment of prisoners. Requires reporting suspected, untreated prisoners upon release to a local health officer. Requires prison medical staff to adhere to current STD medical protocol. Requires the prison to inform the Division of Public Health when a person infected with or suspected of having an STD is released from prison without appropriate treatment, counseling or examination. Allows the division to examine medical records or other medical information to ensure that appropriate STD medical practices are followed. Requires all state, county and city prisons to provide a space necessary to quarantine any person known or suspected of having an STD.

FL   **Fla. Stat. Ann. § 384.27 (West 1993 and Supplemental 1998)** outlines the procedures for physical examinations and treatment of STDs. Specifies that no person can be apprehended, examined or treated for STDs against his or her will, except upon court order. States that the suspected STD-infected person receive written notice within 72 hours of the court order requiring the person to receive treatment. Requires the department to provide clear and convincing evidence that a threat to public health exists when petitioning the court for an order. Allows the court to require counseling and periodic testing for the suspected STD-infected person.

FL   **Fla. Stat. Ann. § 384.28 (West 1993 and Supplemental 1998)** requires specific protocol be followed when attempting hospitalization, placement and treatment for an STD-infected person who is considered a threat to the public health. Allows the department to petition a court order for the hospitalization and treatment of an infected person. Prohibits placing a person under 18 into a hospital or in another health care facility where adults are hospitalized.

FL   **Fla. Stat. Ann. § 384.281 (West 1993 and Supplemental 1998)** provides the department with guidelines for prehearing detention for an STD-infected person who is considered a threat to public health. Outlines procedures for confining an infected person. Requires an infected person to have a bail hearing within 24 hours.

FL   **Fla. Stat. Ann. § 384.284 (West 1993)** requires the department to develop and supply all necessary forms to be used by the circuit court for ordering the physical examination, treatment and hospitalization of an STD-infected person.

FL   **Fla. Stat. Ann. § 384.286 (West 1993)** allows for temporary leave from hospitalization for an STD-infected person for therapeutic reasons or when a death occurs.

GA   **Ga. Code Ann. § 31-17-3 (1996)** authorizes agents of the department to examine any person infected or suspected of being infected with a venereal disease. Authorizes the agent to require the infected person to report for treatment and continue treatment as necessary. Requires law enforcement to assist agents in locating, restraining and arresting any person infected or suspected of being infected with a venereal disease.

ID   **Idaho Code § 39-603 (1993)** authorizes any state, county and municipal health officer to investigate and examine any person reasonably suspected of being infected with a venereal disease and requires that person to report for quarantine and treatment. Requires all local and state health officers to cooperate with proper officials who enforce prostitution laws to control venereal diseases.

ID   **Idaho Code § 39-605 (1993)** authorizes the state Board of Health and Welfare to make rules concerning the control, treatment and quarantine of persons infected with a venereal disease.

IL   **Ill. Ann. Stat. ch. 410 § 325/5 (Smith-Hurd 1997)** requires the department to adopt rules regarding the authorization of interviews for investigating persons infected or believed to be infected with an STD, and to order a person to submit to an examination and treatment. Requires all information gathered during an investigation be confidential. Makes it a Class A misdemeanor for any person who knowingly discloses any information of any person infected with an STD.

IL   **Ill. Ann. Stat. ch. 410 § 325/6 (Smith-Hurd 1997)** authorizes the department to examine any person believed to be infected with an STD. Requires any person believed to be infected with an STD to submit to treatment. Prohibits any person from being apprehended, examined or treated for an STD without a warrant.

IL   **Ill. Ann. Stat. ch. 410 § 325/7 (Smith-Hurd 1997)** authorizes the department to quarantine and isolate any person suspected of being infected with an STD when he or she is a danger to the public health. States that no person may be quarantined or ordered into isolation except with the consent of the person or by court order.

IA   **Iowa Code § 140.8 (1997)** authorizes the local board of health to examine any person reasonably suspected of having a venereal disease in an infectious state. Allows the local board to apply to the court for an order for that person to submit to venereal disease examination. Requires that in every case of treatment ordered by the court, a doctor must certify that the person is no longer infectious.

LA   **La. Rev. Stat. Ann § 1063 (West 1992)** authorizes the department to give an examination to any person suspected of being infected with a venereal disease. Prohibits any person from failing or refusing to submit to an examination for a venereal disease.

LA   **La. Rev. Stat. Ann § 1064 (West 1992)** requires any person infected with a venereal disease to be subject to a quarantine and submit to treatment for the venereal disease by order of the department.

MA   **Mass. Gen. Laws Ann. ch. 111, § 121 (West 1996)** requires any inmate or prisoner who is in a penal institute and who is infected with a venereal disease be isolated and placed under medical treatment. Requires that prison authorities notify the department of the medical care. Requires any prisoner infected with a venereal disease or tuberculosis at the time of prison release be quarantined and treated at public expense. Requires a notice of the prisoner's release be reported to the department. Requires the expenses for the treatment be paid by the town in which the penal institute is situated or, when a state prison, requires the expenses be charged to the state.

MS   **Miss. Code Ann. § 41-23-27 (1993)** authorizes the state Board of Health to isolate, quarantine and treat a person infected with an STD. Authorizes the board to pass rules and regulations regarding isolation, quarantine, confinement and treatment. Makes it a misdemeanor for any person violating any rule or regulation made by the state Board of Health, is punishable by a fine, imprisonment or both.

MS   **Miss. Code Ann. § 41-23-29 (1993)** requires any person suspected of being infected with an STD be subject to an examination and inspection by the state Board of Health. Failure or refusal to be examined may be a misdemeanor.

MT   **Mont. Code Ann. § 50-18-107 (1997)** outlines powers and duties of health officers. Authorizes health officers to examine, isolate or investigate a person suspected of being infected with an STD. Allows only a local or state health officer to terminate a quarantine.

NH   **N.H. Rev. Stat. Ann. § 141-C:18 (1996)** authorizes the director of health to request examination, isolation, quarantine and treatment of any person suspected of having been exposed to or exposing another person to an STD.

NJ   **N.J. Stat. Ann. § 26:4-30 (West 1996)** authorizes the local board or health officer to require a person infected with a venereal disease to submit to an examination.

NJ   **N.J. Stat. Ann. § 26:4-31 (West 1996)** requires a person who is requested by the local board or health officer to submit to an examination and be tested for venereal disease. Requires a person infected with a venereal disease to be examined by a physician of the same sex when requested by the infected person.

NJ   **N.J. Stat. Ann. § 26:4-32 (West 1996)** requires a prostitute or other "lewd" person be considered a person suspected of being infected with a venereal disease and be required to submit to an examination at any time. Requires no certificate of freedom from a venereal disease be issued to any prostitute.

NJ   **N.J. Stat. Ann. § 26:4-35 (West 1996)** allows for isolating and quarantining any person with a venereal disease in an infectious stage who fails to report to a physician .

NJ   **N.J. Stat. Ann. § 26:4-36 (West 1996)** authorizes quarantining a person with a venereal disease when the infected person fails to report to an examination or treatment, or is likely to infect another person with a venereal disease. Requires the quarantine continue until the person is free from the disease.

NJ   **N.J. Stat. Ann. § 26:4-37 (West 1996)** allows a health officer, state commissioner of health or authorized representative to file a complaint with the court when a venereal disease-infected person fails or refuses to comply with a quarantine.

NJ   **N.J. Stat. Ann. § 26:4-48 (West 1996)** requires the state department to make and enforce any rule or regulation for quarantining and treating a person with a venereal disease. Requires the state director or other official persons to have the power to quarantine an infected person, and to require or request examinations or treatment for an STD-infected person.

NJ   **N.J. Stat. Ann. § 26:4-48.1 (West 1996)** allows a person infected with a venereal disease who is quarantined be exempt from treatment due to religious principles.

NJ   **N.J. Stat. Ann. § 26:4-49.7 (West 1996)** requires the court to order a person who is suspected of being infected with a venereal disease and who is coming before the court on any charge to submit to an examination and treatment.

NJ   **N.J. Stat. Ann. § 26:4-49.8 (West 1996)** requires examining and treating a prisoner for a venereal disease. Allows a prisoner be isolated when a prisoner refuses treatment for a venereal disease. Requires the warden to notify the department when a prisoner with a venereal disease will be released. Requires the notification to be five days prior to the actual date of release or no later than the day following the release date.

NM   **N. M. Stat. Ann. § 30-9-5 (1994)** allows the court to order a venereal disease examination and treatment for a person convicted of prostitution or soliciting a prostitute. Requires the state to pay for medical treatment when the infected person is unable to pay.

NY   **N.Y. Public Health Law § 2300 (McKinney 1993)** allows a health officer to require a medical examination for STD infection and to determine at which stage the infection is communicable. Requires the person submit to an examination and, if the person refuses, he or she shall be isolated. Outlines the examination procedure. Requires the physician making the exam to report promptly to the health officer and prohibits issuing a certificate of freedom from STDs to the person examined.

NY   **N.Y. Public Health Law § 2301 (McKinney 1993)** allows a health officer to apply to court for an order to examine a person who is refusing to be tested for an STD. Requires all papers pertaining to any proceedings be kept confidential except to those authorized to inspect the report.

NY   **N.Y. Public Health Law § 2302 (McKinney 1993)** requires any person arrested for failure to comply with a court order for an STD examination, or arrested for frequenting houses of prostitution be examined for STDs. Outlines court procedures. Prohibits the release of any person convicted until that person has been examined.

NY   **N.Y. Public Health Law § 2303 (McKinney 1993)** allows a health officer to require a person to submit to treatment or isolation if the person is found to be infected with an STD in a stage that may become communicable. Requires the health officer to define the place and limits of the isolation area and when isolation may be terminated.

ND   **N.D. Cent. Code § 23-07-07 (1991)** authorizes the state, local and city health officers, when necessary for the protection of public health, to examine any person suspected of being infected with an STD, to require any person to report for treatment, and to investigate any cases and cooperate with other officials to enforce the laws.

ND   **N.D. Cent. Code § 23-07-09 (1991)** requires prison authorities of any state, county or city prison to make available a portion of the prison for isolating and treating a person infected with an STD.

ND   **N.D. Cent. Code § 23-07.7-01 (1997)** allows the court to order any defendant or any alleged juvenile offender charged with a sex offense to submit to medical testing for STDs. Allows the court to order the testing only if the court receives a petition from the alleged victim. Requires a copy of the test results be released to the defendant's or alleged juvenile offender's physician and each requesting victim's physician. Outlines court procedures.

ND   **N.D. Cent. Code § 23-07.7-02 (1997)** outlines testing procedures for court-ordered testing. Requires testing for HIV and STDs. Requires laboratory to send a copy of test results to the physician who supplies results to defendant and victim, and the department. Makes it a Class C felony for any person who violates confidentiality.

OH   **Ohio Rev. Code Ann. § 3709.24 (Page 1997)** allows a board of health of any city or general health district to set up clinics to provide free treatment for gonorrhea, syphilis and chancroid. Allows these clinics to be used for quarantining cases of gonorrhea, syphilis and chancroid or other cases the director of health orders to be quarantined.

OK   **Okla. Stat. Ann. tit. 63, § 1-518 (1997)** makes it unlawful for any STD-infected person to refuse, fail or neglect to report to an examination and treatment by a physician.

OK   **Okla. Stat. Ann. tit. 63, § 1-524 (1997)** requires examining all prisoners to determine if a prisoner is infected with an STD. Allows a licensed physician to examine persons who are arrested for prostitution or other sex crimes. Allows for a person to be detained until the results are known. Requires any person found to be infected with an STD to be treated. Requires quarantining any person who refuses treatment. Requires a person who is arrested for rape and other serious sexual crimes be tested for STDs and HIV. Authorizes the court to issue an order for testing during the arraignment. Requires the order not to include the name and address of the alleged victim. Requires the alleged victim be notified of the test results.

OK   **Okla. Stat. Ann. tit. 63, § 1-530 (1997)** requires a local health officer, upon hearing a case of a venereal disease, authorize a quarantine of the person infected with a venereal disease. Requires the state board of health to adopt rules and regulations for quarantining an infected person.

PA   **Pa. Cons. Stat. Ann. tit. 35, § 521.8 (Purdon 1993)** authorizes a local health officer to require any person suspected of being infected with a venereal disease to be examined and treated. Allows the health officer to quarantine any person who refuses treatment. Allows the health officer to file a court petition stating the person is suspected of being infected with a venereal disease.

PA   **Pa. Cons. Stat. Ann. tit. 35, § 521.8 (Purdon 1993)** allows any person taken into custody and charged with a sex offense crime to be examined for a venereal disease by a department or court-appointed physician. Allows any person convicted of a crime and suspected of being infected to be examined for a venereal disease. Requires treating any person found to be infected with a venereal disease.

PA   **Pa. Cons. Stat. Ann. tit. 35, § 521.11 (Purdon 1993)** allows any local health officer to quarantine any person infected with a venereal disease who refuses treatment. Allow the secretary or local health officer to file a court petition to commit the infected person to the appropriate institution or hospital. Allows for the religious treatment as long as the quarantine requirement is kept. Allows the department to use any county jail for isolating the infected person during treatment. Requires the local board or department to reimburse the institution for use of treating the infected person.

RI   **R.I. Gen. Laws § 23-11-3 (1996)** authorizes the department to require a person who is infected with an STD to report for treatment and continue treatment until cured. Requires anyone who refuses treatment to be isolated.

RI   **R.I. Gen. Laws § 23-11-11 (1996)** authorizes the department to examine any person reasonably suspected of having an STD. Requires the department to inform the infected person of the right to have his or her own physician present. Allows any person under age 18 to give consent for the examination and treatment of an STD. Releases the physician examining the minor from any liability.

SC   **S.C. Code Ann. § 44-29-90 (Law. Co-op 1997)** authorizes state, district, county and municipal health officers to examine, isolate and treat any person infected or suspected of being infected with an STD. Requires an infected person report for treatment at public expense. Requires the infected person to identify anyone with whom they have had sexual contact, intravenous drug use, or both. Makes available state resources to be used when a person is identified as being infected with HIV/AIDS and has known sexual contacts, intravenous drug use contacts, or both. Requires notifying anyone who may have been infected and also requires the identity of the person who infected them not be revealed.

SC   **S.C. Code Ann. § 44-29-100 (Law. Co-op 1997)** authorizes health authorities to examine or treat any person who is imprisoned in any state, county or city prison. Requires a person, who after serving his or her sentence, is suffering from an STD, be isolated and treated at public expense. Allows a person to report for treatment to a licensed physician at public expense.

SC   **S.C. Code Ann. § 44-29-110 (Law. Co-op 1997)** requires a person suffering from an STD not be discharged from quarantine unless authorized by a state, county or municipal health officer.

SD   **S.D. Codified Laws Ann. § 34-23-4 (1994)** allows any state, county and municipal health officer to require an infected person with a venereal disease to report for treatment. Allows an officer to quarantine an infected person.

SD   **S.D. Codified Laws Ann. § 34-23-5 (1994)** authorizes quarantining or isolating any person who is convicted of being a prostitute and who also is infected with a venereal disease.

SD   **S.D. Codified Laws Ann. § 34-23-7 (1994)** allows health authorities to use any state, county or city prison for isolating and treating a prisoner with a venereal disease.

SD   **S.D. Codified Laws Ann. § 34-23-13 (1994)** requires the state department to make rules and regulations concerning the care, treatment and quarantine of persons infected with a venereal disease.

TN   **Tenn. Code Ann. § 68-10-104 (1996)** authorizes state, district, county and municipal health officers to investigate and examine any person reasonably suspected of being infected with an STD, and requires such person to report for treatment and quarantine. Allows any state, district, county or municipal health officer or any physician to examine, diagnose and treat minors infected with an STD without the knowledge or consent of the parents. Releases the physician or health officer from any liability except for negligence.

TN   **Tenn. Code Ann. § 68-10-105 (1996)** authorizes a health officer to designate and define limits within a specified area where the STD-infected person is to be isolated or quarantined. Authorizes only the physician or nurse working on the case to enter or leave the area of quarantine without the permission of the health officer.

TN   **Tenn. Code Ann. § 68-10-106 (1996)** requires that no one but a state, municipal, district or county health officer establish and terminate the quarantine of persons infected with STDs. Requires the commissioner to set up clinical laboratory criteria for the guidance of health officers in the performance of their duties regarding quarantining an infected person.

TN   **Tenn. Code Ann. § 68-10-108 (1996)** authorizes county legislative bodies, city officials and other boards to provide a place for the isolation and quarantine of an STD-infected person.

TN   **Tenn. Code Ann. § 68-10-109 (1996)** authorizes the department to make rules and bylaws for the control of STDs, including the reporting, isolation and quarantining of STD-infected persons.

TN   **Tenn. Code Ann. § 68-10-110 (1996)** allows a health officer to appeal to the court for an arrest of a person infected with an STD who refuses treatment. Outlines court procedures for the arrest and temporary commitment for treatment. Requires the examination be made by a health officer or licensed and practicing physician. Allows the infected person to have his or her own physician present at the exam. Allows for an appeal by the infected person.

UT   **Utah Code Ann. § 26-6-17 (1995)** authorizes any state, county or municipal health officer to examine any person reasonably suspected of being infected with a venereal disease. Requires a person infected with a venereal disease to report for treatment and continue treatment until cured. Requires treatment be provided at the public's expense when the infected person is unable to pay.

VT   **Vt. Stat. Ann. tit. 18, § 1092 (1982)** requires any physician or other qualified person providing medical care to a person infected with gonorrhea or syphilis to report the case to the state. Requires the infected person submit to treatment until discharged by a physician. Stipulates that any person who refuses treatment be reported to the state and punished by a fine of no more than $100, or three months in prison, or both.

VT   **Vt. Stat. Ann. tit. 18, § 1093 (1982)** authorizes the board to require any person reasonably suspected of being infected with a venereal disease to undergo a medical exam and testing by a licensed physician. Allows for the suspected person to be detained until the results are known. Requires the physician to report the test results to the board.

VT   **Vt. Stat. Ann. tit. 18, § 1100 (1982)** requires the board to make and enforce any rule or regulation for quarantining and treating any reported venereal disease cases for the protection of the public.

VA   **Va. Code § 32.1-57 (1997)** allows a local health director to require any person suspected of being infected with any venereal disease to submit to an examination, testing and treatment. Allows the local health director to apply to the court for any order if the person refuses to submit to an examination, testing or treatment, or fails to continue treatment. Requires treatment be free of charge when an infected person with a venereal disease is required by the local health director to receive treatment.

WA   **Wash. Rev. Code Ann. § 70.24.022 (1996)** requires the board to adopt rules authorizing interviews of all persons infected with an STD, to investigate the source, and to order an infected or believed to be infected person to submit to an examination, counseling and treatment. Requires all information gathered to be held confidential. Allows a person who is reasonably believed to be infected with an STD to reveal the name or names of sexual contacts and not be held liable. Makes it a gross misdemeanor for any person who knowingly gives any false information concerning the existence of any STD.

WA   **Wash. Rev. Code Ann. § 70.24.024 (1996)** authorizes state and local health officers or other authorized persons to examine any person believed to be infected or exposed to an STD. Authorizes a health officer to order a person to submit to a medical examination, testing, counseling or treatment within 14 days of the initial investigation. Authorizes a health officer to restrict a person from any behavior or conduct that endangers the public. Requires these restrictions be in writing. Outlines issuance of the restriction order and court proceedings. Requires all information be confidential unless a public hearing is requested.

WA   **Wash. Rev. Code Ann. § 70.24.070 (1996)** authorizes the board to designate facilities for the detention and treatment of a person infected with an STD. Allows any facility in any hospital or other public or private institution, other than a jail or correctional facility, to be used to segregate, isolate and treat an infected person.

WA   **Wash. Rev. Code Ann. § 70.24.105 (Supplemental 1997)** prohibits any person to disclose or be compelled to disclose the identity of any person who has investigated, considered or requested a test or treatment for an STD. Allows the exchange of medical information with certain authorized medical and social services personnel and law enforcement officers, or by court order. Allows disclosure of test results upon the request of a victim of a sex crime.

WV   **W. Va. Code § 16-4-3 (1995)** authorizes any municipal or county health officer to establish a medical clinic for the use of the detention and quarantine of a person infected with a venereal disease.

WV   **W. Va. Code § 16-4-9 (1995)** requires a physician or other person who examines or treats a person with syphilis, gonorrhea or chancroid to inform that person of the necessity of taking treatment and continuing the treatment as prescribed. Requires a physician to report a patient who has stopped treatment to the local health officer. Makes it a misdemeanor for anyone to stop treatment for a venereal disease. Requires the local health officer to investigate any unfinished treatments for a venereal disease. Authorizes the local health officer to arrest, detain and quarantine any patient who fails to return for treatment.

WV   **W. Va. Code § 16-4-12 (1995)** allows a local health officer to investigate, arrest, detain and quarantine any person who is suffering from a venereal disease in an infectious stage and is not under treatment.

WV   **W. Va. Code § 16-4-21 (1995)** authorizes a health officer to establish a quarantine for a person infected with a venereal disease. Makes it a misdemeanor for anyone who does not follow the health officer's quarantining rules.

WI   **Wis. Stat. Ann. § 252.10 (West Supplemental 1997)** requires a physician to notify the department when an STD-infected person refuses or stops treatment. Authorizes the department to take the necessary steps to have the person committed for treatment or observation. Allows the court to commit to treatment persons who refuse. Outlines court procedures.

WY   **Wyo. Stat. § 35-4-133 (1997)** authorizes a health officer to isolate and examine an STD-infected or suspected to be an infected individual. Requires the individual to submit to treatment at public expense. Allows providing STD education information and counseling for the STD-infected individual. Requires the health officer to notify any person who may have been exposed. Requires the health officer to investigate sources of STDs and cooperate with the proper law enforcement in enforcing the laws against prostitution.

WY   **Wyo. Stat. § 35-4-134 (1997)** authorizes a health officer to examine, treat and isolate a prisoner confined at any state, county or city jail. Requires providing minimum care and treatment of the individual infected with an incurable STD. Requires examination and treatment of prisoners.

Reporting—Gonorrhea

AR   **Ark. Stat. Ann. § 20-16-501 (1991)** requires a laboratory to report to the department any positive tests of syphilis, gonorrhea, chancroid and other reportable venereal diseases.

IA   **Iowa Code § 140.5 (1997)** requires any person in charge of a public or private laboratory to report any positive tests for syphilis, gonorrhea, chancroid, granuloma inguinale or lymphogranuloma venereum. Requires that the report have the name of the person being tested, the name and address of the physician or other person submitting the specimen, the lab results and the date.

NC   **N.C. Gen. Stat. § 130A-139 (1997)** requires a person in charge of a laboratory to report any positive gonorrhea, syphilis or tuberculosis test.

OH   **Ohio Rev. Code Ann. § 3701.46 (Page 1997)** requires a physician or other required medical personnel to report on the birth or fetal death certificate that blood tests for syphilis and gonorrhea were performed on the mother and approximate dates of the tests. Prohibits the results of the tests be stated on the birth or fetal death certificate.

OH   **Ohio Rev. Code Ann. § 3701.48 (Page 1997)** requires a laboratory making the standard tests for syphilis and gonorrhea to give a report to the physician or health commissioner who submits the specimens. Requires laboratories to report any reactive syphilis test or positive gonorrhea test to the department.

VT   **Vt. Stat. Ann. tit. 18, § 1092 (1982)** requires any physician or other qualified person providing medical care to a person infected with gonorrhea or syphilis to report the case to the state. Requires the infected person submit to treatment until discharged by a physician. Stipulates that any person who refuses treatment be reported to the state and punished by a fine of no more than $100, or three months in prison, or both.

WV   **W. Va. Code § 16-4-6 (1995)** requires any physician, hospital or penal institution to report a diagnosis or treatment of a syphilis, gonorrhea or charoid case to the local municipal health officer and to the director of health.

WV   **W. Va. Code § 16-4-11 (1995)** requires a physician to report and to notify the local health officer of any person who is suspected of having syphilis, gonorrhea or chancroid and is exposing others to the infection. Requires the local health officer to investigate any suspected venereal disease cases.

Reporting—Other

AL   **Ala. Code § 22-11A-13 (1997)** authorizes and directs the Board of Health to declare rules for testing, reporting, investigation and treatment of STDs.

AL   **Ala. Code § 22-11A-14 (1997)** outlines reporting procedures for STDs. Requires a physician who diagnoses or treats STDs to report to the state or county health officer. Requires laboratories to report all positive or reactive STD tests. Requires all reports and documentation be confidential. Makes it a misdemeanor for violating any reporting rules with a penalty ranging from $100 to $500 upon conviction.

AK   **Alaska Stat. § 18.15.310** requires that all blood drawn for a court-ordered HIV or STD test of a person charged with a sex offense be performed by a physician, physician's assistant or other qualified personnel and tested in a medically approved laboratory. Requires all test results that indicate exposure to or infection by HIV or other STDs be reported to the department. Requires anyone who receives test results, other than the test subjects, maintain confidentiality. Requires the department provide free counseling and free testing to the victim for HIV and other STDs and counseling to the alleged sex offender upon request of the offender. Requires the department to provide referral to appropriate health care facilities and support services at the request of the victim.

AR   **Ark. Stat. Ann. § 20-16-501 (1991)** requires a laboratory to report any positive tests of syphilis, gonorrhea, chancroid and other reportable venereal diseases to the department.

AR   **Ark. Stat. Ann. § 20-16-502 (1991)** outlines reporting process for a positive venereal disease test result. Requires that when notifying the department about a positive or doubtful test result, the report must contain the name, age, sex and address of the infected person, name of the test performed and the date of the test.

AR   **Ark. Stat. Ann. § 20-16-503 (1991)** requires a physician to report any venereal disease cases to the department.

AR   **Ark. Stat. Ann. § 20-16-505 (1991)** authorizes the department to make rules and regulations relating to the reporting procedure for a venereal disease.

AR   **Ark. Stat. Ann. § 20-16-506 (1991)** makes it a misdemeanor for any physician or laboratory to fail to report a venereal disease with a punishable fine of no less than $10 and no more than $20.

CA   **Cal. Health & Safety Code § 120590-605 (West 1996)** requires the county district attorney to prosecute any person accused of violating the investigation, rules and regulations of reporting or treating a person with STDs.

CA   **Cal. Health & Safety Code § 120700 (West 1996)** requires a laboratory to submit the report of records to the department when required by the department. Allows reports to be destroyed after two years.

CA   **Cal. Health & Safety Code § 125085 (West 1996)** requires a blood specimen of a pregnant woman be submitted to an approved public health lab to determine the presence of Hepatitis B. Requires the test results be reported to the attending physician and the woman tested.

CO   **Colo. Rev. Stat. § 25-4-402 (1997)** requires any physician, intern or other person who makes a venereal disease diagnosis to report the case to the health authorities.

CT   **Conn. Gen. Stat. § 54-102a (1997)** allows a court to order persons charged with certain sexual offenses to undergo a venereal examination and HIV testing. Requires reporting the results to the department. Allows the court to order treatment if HIV or a venereal disease is found. Requires the examination or test be paid for by the department. Makes it a Class C misdemeanor for any person who fails to comply with any court-ordered testing or treatment.

DE   **Del. Code Ann. tit. 16, § 702 (1996)** outlines the reporting procedures for STDs. Requires any physician who diagnoses or treats STDs to report to the state or county health officer. Requires any lab that conducts STD testing report all positive or reactive tests. Requires all reports and documentation be held confidential. Authorizes the state or county to follow appropriate procedures for infection control.

DE   **Del. Code Ann. tit. 16, § 707 (1996)** authorizes the department to make rules and regulations in regard to reporting, controlling and treating people with STDs.

FL   **Fla. Stat. Ann. § 384.25 (West 1998)** requires any person who violates the reporting procedures or does not maintain confidentiality to be fined up to $500 for each offense. Requires the department to report each violation to the regulatory agency responsible for licensing health care professionals and laboratories.

FL   **Fla. Stat. Ann. § 385.25 (West 1998)** requires any person who diagnoses a person with an STD and any laboratory that conducts a positive STD test result to report the diagnosis to the department within two weeks. Requires the department to adopt rules specifying the information required and a minimum time period for reporting STDs. Requires the department to consider the need for information, privacy and confidentiality of the patient, and the practical ability of authorized personnel and labs to report in a reasonable fashion.

GA   **Ga. Code Ann. § 31-17-2 (1996)** requires a physician or other person who makes a diagnosis or treats a venereal case, or any manager of a hospital or penal institution, to report any venereal disease case to the health authorities.

GA   **Ga. Code Ann. § 31-17-6 (1996)** requires all laboratories conducting venereal disease tests to comply with the rules, regulations and reporting requirements prescribed by the department.

HI   **Hawaii Rev. Stat. § 325-52 (1993)** outlines serologic testing and reporting. Requires requested tests to be free of charge when completed at a department laboratory. Requires the department to issue a "laboratory report form." Outlines the procedure for reporting.

ID   **Idaho Code § 39-602 (1993)** requires any physician; manager of a hospital, dispensary, charitable or penal institution; or other person who makes a diagnosis or treats a venereal disease to report the case to the department.

ID   **Idaho Code § 39-1004 (1993)** provides guidelines in reporting laboratory tests. Requires laboratories to furnish a detailed report and result of the serological syphilis test. Requires a laboratory not operated by the department to file a report with the department. Maintains that reports are kept confidential and not open for public inspection.

IL   **Ill. Ann. Stat. ch. 410 § 325/4 (Smith-Hurd 1997)** outlines the reporting procedures for STDs. Requires any physician who diagnoses or treats STDs to report to the state or county health officer. Requires any laboratory that conducts STD testing report all positive or reactive tests. Makes it a Class A misdemeanor for any person who provides false information. Imposes $500 fine on any person who violates the rules of the department. Requires the department to report each violation to the regulatory agency responsible for licensing a health care professional or a laboratory.

IN   **Ind. Code Ann. § 16-41-14-9 (Burns 1993)** requires a practitioner to report the name and address of a semen donor or recipient to the department if an STD or HIV is present. Requires a practitioner to attempt to notify a donor or recipient if the semen tested is positive for STD or HIV. Requires reporting of the test results.

IA   **Iowa Code § 140.4 (1997)** requires reporting immediately after the first examination or treatment any person infected with any venereal disease. Requires the report to include the name, age, sex, marital status, occupation of patient, name of the disease, probable source of infection and duration of the disease. Requires that reports be confidential. Requires immunity from any civil or criminal liability for any person making a report.

IA   **Iowa Code § 140.5 (1997)** requires any person in charge of a public or private laboratory to report any positive tests for syphilis, gonorrhea, chancroid, granuloma inguinale or lymphogranuloma venereum. Requires that the report have the name of the person being tested, the name and address of the physician or other person submitting the specimen, the lab results and the date.

IA   **Iowa Code § 140.6 (1997)** makes it a simple misdemeanor for any physician or other person who is required to report a venereal disease who does not report or falsely reports any information concerning an STD-infected person, or who discloses the identity of that person. Requires that failure to report a venereal disease as specified may result in the refusal of a license renewal.

LA   **La. Rev. Stat. Ann § 1065 (West 1992)** requires a licensed physician or manager of a hospital to report any venereal disease case to the department. Requires the report be made within 24 hours after the case has first been diagnosed. Requires a physician to report a person infected with the venereal disease for failing or refusing, for a period of 10 days or more after the diagnosis, to submit to treatment. Requires a physician to report when an infected person exposes another person to a venereal disease infection.

LA   **La. Rev. Stat. Ann § 1067 (West 1992)** requires the secretary of the department to make rules and regulations for the diagnosis, treatment, reporting and prevention of venereal diseases.

94

MA   **Mass. Gen. Laws Ann. ch. 111, § 121 (West 1996)** requires any inmate or prisoner in a penal institute infected with a venereal disease be isolated and placed under medical treatment. Requires that prison authorities notify the department of the medical care. Requires any prisoner infected with a venereal disease or tuberculosis at the time of prison release be quarantined and treated at public expense. Requires a notice of the prisoner's release be reported to the department. Requires the expenses for the treatment be paid by the town in which the penal institute is located or, when a state prison, requires the expenses be charged to the state.

MI   **Mich. Stat. Ann. § 14.15 (5111) (Law. Co-op 1995)** authorizes the department to establish reporting requirements for serious communicable diseases. Allows the department to require a licensed health professional or health facility to report a serious communicable disease or infection within 24 hours of diagnosis. Requires local health departments to furnish care for tuberculosis and venereal diseases. Requires the department to provide rules for the confidentiality of reports, records and data pertaining to the testing, care, treatment, reporting and research associated with tuberculosis, Hepatitis B and other venereal diseases.

MI   **Mich. Stat. Ann. § 14.15 (Law. Co-op 1995)** requires the local health department to provide medical care for any person with a serious communicable disease or infection including tuberculosis and any venereal disease. Requires the local department to report the case to the individual's county department of social services.

MT   **Mont. Code Ann. § 50-19-105 (1997)** requires all positive tests for STDs be reported to the department by the laboratory preparing the test.

NE   **Neb. Rev. Stat. § 71-502.04 (1996)** outlines reporting procedures. Requires each report supply date, name, result of test performed and, when available, age of the person. Requires name and address of physician requesting test. Requires all laboratory reports be held confidential and not open to public inspection with certain exceptions.

NJ   **N.J. Stat. Ann. § 26:4-38 (West 1996)** requires any physician, nurse or other person treating a venereal disease to report the case to the state department.

NJ   **N.J. Stat. Ann. § 26:4-39 (West 1996)** requires any state, county or municipal hospital, mental institution, or public or private institution to report any cases of venereal disease to the state department.

NM   **N. M. Stat. Ann. § 24-1-7 (1997)** requires a physician or manager of a clinic who makes diagnosis, treats or prescribes for an STD case, or a laboratory with a positive STD test, to report the case immediately to the district health officer. Requires all district health officers to make weekly reports to the department of all STD cases reported during the preceding week.

NY   **N.Y. Public Health Law § 2300 (McKinney 1993)** allows a health officer to require a medical examination for STD infection and to determine at which stage the infection is communicable. Requires the person submit to an examination, and if the person refuses, he or she shall be isolated. Outlines the examination procedure. Requires the physician making the exam to report promptly to the health officer and not issue a certificate of freedom from STDs to the person examined.

NY   **N.Y. Public Health Law § 2309 (McKinney 1993)** makes it a misdemeanor for any person who violates the rules and regulations of the department regarding testing, reporting and confidentiality of STDs.

NC   **N.C. Gen. Stat. § 15A-615 (1997)** allows testing a sex offender who has had an alleged sexual contact with any minor under age 16 for STDs, including chlamydia, gonorrhea, Hepatitis B, herpes, HIV and syphilis. Allows the victim to petition the court for the offender to be tested. Requires the test results be reported to the local health director. Requires the victim and alleged offender be informed of the tests results and be provided with counseling. Requires the results of the test not be admissible as evidence in any criminal proceeding.

ND   **N.D. Cent. Code § 23-07-03 (1997)** requires the superintendent of a hospital, dispensary, or charitable or penal institution to report any cases of STDs to the nearest health officer.

OK   **Okla. Stat. Ann. tit. 63, § 1-527 (1997)** requires a physician who makes a diagnosis or treats a venereal disease case, or any manager of a hospital or prison who is aware of a venereal disease case, to report the case immediately to the state commissioner of health.

OK   **Okla. Stat. Ann. tit. 63, § 1-528 (1997)** requires a physician who examines or treats a person with a venereal disease to instruct the infected person on how to prevent the spread of the disease and the necessity for treatment. Requires a physician or other person who suspects a person who has a venereal disease is exposing others to the infection to notify the local health officer.

PR	**P.R. Laws Ann. tit. 24, § 572 (1993)** requires the lab to report within five days along with the name of patient, age, sex, address and name of the doctor. Mandates all report remain confidential.
PR	**P.R. Laws Ann. tit. 24, § 574 (1993)** requires doctors to notify the department of STD cases within five days.
PR	**P.R. Laws Ann. tit. 24, § 575 (1993)** states that it is the civic responsibility of laboratories and doctors to report their findings.
RI	**R.I. Gen. Laws § 23-11-5 (1996)** requires a superintendent or any other person in charge of public or private institutions to promptly report the identity of any patients in his or her heir care who is suffering from an STD.
RI	**R.I. Gen. Laws § 23-11-6 (1996)** requires a physician who diagnoses and treats an STD case to report the case to the state department.
RI	**R.I. Gen. Laws § 23-11-7 (1996)** requires a penalty for failure to report an STD case. Requires any superintendent, physician or other who fails to report an STD case within a 10-day period of first knowing about the case be fined no more than $100.
RI	**R.I. Gen. Laws § 23-11-14 (1996)** requires any public or private laboratory performing a test for an STD to report the result, reactive or positive, within 10 days of the test.
SC	**S.C. Code Ann. § 44-29-70 (Law. Co-op 1997)** requires any physician or other person who makes a diagnosis or treats an STD case to report it to the health authorities.
SC	**S.C. Code Ann. § 44-29-80 (Law. Co-op 1997)** requires laboratories to report positive STD test results.
SC	**S.C. Code Ann. § 44-29-135 (Law. Co-op 1997)** requires information not be released or made public except with the written consent of persons identified. Allows information to be released for statistical purposes where the individual cannot be identified, and for medical information necessary to enforce the control and treatment of STDs and protect the health of the STD-infected person. Requires reporting the name and the medical information of a minor with no further information required to be released by the department.
SD	**S.D. Codified Laws Ann. § 34-23-2 (1994)** requires a physician or other person who diagnoses or treats a person with a venereal disease to report the case to the department. Requires the identity of the infected individual in the report and investigation be kept confidential and not disclosed to any court.
TN	**Tenn. Code Ann. § 68-10-101 (1996)** requires physicians, health officers, clinics, hospitals, labs or penal institutions to report any STD cases. Outlines reporting procedures.
TN	**Tenn. Code Ann. § 68-10-109 (1996)** authorizes the department to make rules and bylaws for the control of STDs, including the reporting, isolation and quarantining of STD-infected persons.
VT	**Vt. Stat. Ann. tit. 18, § 1093 (1982)** authorizes the board to require any person reasonably suspected of being infected with a venereal disease to undergo a medical exam and testing by a licensed physician. Allows the suspected person to be detained until the results are known. Requires the physician to report the test results to the board.
VT	**Vt. Stat. Ann. tit. 18, § 1101 (1982)** requires any superintendent or person in charge of any public institution, hospital, dispensary, clinic or correctional institution to report to the state any patient suffering from a venereal disease.
VA	**Va. Code § 32.1-36 (1997)** requires a physician who diagnoses a venereal disease in a child age 12 or younger to report the case to the authorities, unless the physician reasonably believes that the infection was acquired congenitally or by means other than sexual abuse. Requires all information reported be confidential.
VA	**Va. Code § 32.1-59 (1997)** requires any person admitted to any state correctional institution or state hospital to be examined and tested for a venereal disease. Requires the institution to provide treatment and report the case.
WA	**Wash. Rev. Code Ann. § 70.24.125 (1996)** requires the board to establish reporting requirements for STDs.
WV	**W. Va. Code § 16-4-6 (1995)** requires any physician, hospital or penal institution to report a diagnosis or treatment of a syphilis, gonorrhea or chacroid case to the local municipal health officer and to the director of health.

WV — **W. Va. Code § 16-4-7 (1995)** makes it a misdemeanor for any physician or other person required to make a venereal disease report to fail to report or to make false statements on the report. Allows the medical licensing board to revoke the license of a physician for failing to give or providing false information about a person with a venereal disease.

WV — **W. Va. Code § 16-4-9 (1995)** requires a physician or other person who examines or treats a person with syphilis, gonorrhea or chancroid to inform that person of the necessity of taking treatment and continuing the treatment as prescribed. Requires a physician to report a patient who has stopped treatment to the local health officer. Makes it a misdemeanor for anyone to stop treatment for a venereal disease. Requires the local health officer to investigate any unfinished treatments for a venereal disease. Authorizes the local health officer to arrest, detain and quarantine any patient who fails to return for treatment.

WV — **W. Va. Code § 16-4-11 (1995)** requires a physician to report and to notify the local health officer of any person who is suspected of having syphilis, gonorrhea or chancroid and is exposing others to the infection. Requires the local health officer to investigate any suspected venereal disease cases.

WV — **W. Va. Code § 16-4-18 (1995)** makes it unlawful for any person having a venereal disease in an infectious stage to work at a barbershop, bakery, hotel or restaurant. Requires the physician reporting the venereal disease case to notify the local health officer about the employee. Makes it a misdemeanor for anyone who is infected with a venereal disease who does not stop working within 24 hours.

WI — **Wis. Stat. Ann. § 252.10 (West Supplemental 1997)** requires state laboratories to examine specimens for the diagnosis of STDs for any physician or local health officer in the state. Requires all laboratories to report all positive results to the local health officer and to the department with the name of the physician who diagnosed the case.

WY — **Wyo. Stat. § 7-1-109 (1977)** requires testing for STDs in sexual offense cases. Outlines court procedures. Requires examination results to be reported to the appropriate health officer. Requires the health officer to notify the victim, alleged victim or, if a minor, the parents or guardian of the victim or the alleged victim. Requires costs of any medical examination be funded through the department. Requires all results be held confidential and are not admissible as evidence in court and will not be disclosed except under certain circumstances.

WY — **Wyo. Stat. § 35-4-130 (1997)** makes it a misdemeanor for any person violating or refusing to comply with the rules and regulations regarding STD testing, treatment and reporting, and is punishable by a fine of no more than $750, imprisonment for no more than six months, or both.

WY — **Wyo. Stat. § 35-4-132 (1997)** requires a physician, other health care provider, or administrator of a hospital, dispensary, charitable or penal institution, who diagnoses or treats an STD case to report the diagnosis to the department and the appropriate health officer. Requires all labs with positive laboratory STD tests to report the diseases. Requires health care providers and facilities to cooperate with and assist the department and health officers in preventing the spread of STDs. Requires the department to compile the number of reported cases within the state.

WY — **Wyo. Stat. § 35-4-133 (1997)** allows a health worker to request testing of a person possibly infected with an STD. Allows the county to apply for a court order to have a test performed if the patient does not consent to testing. Requires test results be kept confidential and reported to the state.

Reporting—Syphilis

AL   **Ala. Code § 22-11A-16 (1997)** establishes the procedure for serologic syphilis testing for pregnant women during the first and third trimesters. Requires the samples be submitted to an approved laboratory. Requires testing newborns for syphilis. Requires reporting all positive or reactive tests.

AZ   **Ariz. Rev. Stat. Ann. § 36-694 (1993)** requires a physician to report on the birth or stillbirth certificate that a blood test for syphilis was made either from the mother or from the umbilical cord at the delivery and the approximate date when the specimen was taken.

AR   **Ark. Stat. Ann. § 20-16-501 (1991)** requires a laboratory to report any positive tests of syphilis, gonorrhea, chancroid and other reportable venereal diseases to the department.

AR   **Ark. Stat. Ann. § 20-16-507 (1991)** requires a physician to take a blood sample of a pregnant woman and submit the sample to an approved laboratory for a standard serological test for syphilis. Requires others not allowed by law to take blood but allowed to attend a pregnant woman, to make sure the procedure is completed. Requires tests be free of charge when requested. Requires a physician and others authorized to make reports to state on the birth or stillbirth certificate that a blood sample was taken for a syphilis test and the approximate date.

CO   **Colo. Rev. Stat. § 25-4-203 (1990)** requires a physician to report on the birth or stillbirth certificate that a blood test for syphilis was conducted and the approximate date of the test. Prohibits stating the test result on the birth certificate.

CT   **Conn. Gen. Stat. § 7-61 (1997)** requires a physician or others permitted to report on the birth or fetal death certificate that a blood test for syphilis was made during the pregnancy and the approximate date of the test. Requires stating the reason why a test was not completed. Prohibits stating the test result on the birth certificate.

ID   **Idaho Code § 39-1004 (1993)** provides guidelines in reporting laboratory tests. Requires laboratories to furnish a detailed report and result of the serological syphilis test. Requires a laboratory not operated by the department to file a report with the department. Maintains that reports are kept confidential and not open for public inspection.

IN   **Ind. Code Ann. § 16-41-14-14 (Burns 1997)** requires a practitioner to keep a record of the information of semen used in artificial insemination including any HIV, syphilis or Hepatitis B test results. Allows records kept to be made available to the state department for inspection. Allows the department to enter and inspect a practitioner's facility to investigate the premises, books and records. Prohibits any person from interfering with the performance of the department.

IN   **Ind. Code Ann. § 16-41-15-13 (Burns 1993)** outlines procedures required by the health department for reporting a serological test for syphilis on a birth or stillbirth certificate. Requires the date of the test and whether the test was made during pregnancy or at the time of delivery. Requires stating the reason if the test was not done.

IA   **Iowa Code § 140.5 (1997)** requires any person in charge of a public or private laboratory to report any positive tests for syphilis, gonorrhea, chancroid, granuloma inguinale or lymphogranuloma venereum. Requires that the report have the name of the person being tested, the name and address of the physician or other person submitting the specimen, the lab results and the date.

IA   **Iowa Code § 140.12 (1997)** requires a physician to report on the birth or stillbirth certificate that a blood test for syphilis was made and the approximate date of the test. Requires reporting when the test is not given. Prohibits stating the test result on the birth certificate.

KS   **Kan. Stat. Ann § 65-153f (Supplemental 1997)** requires a physician or a person attending a pregnant woman, with the consent of the woman, to take a blood sample for a serological test for syphilis and Hepatitis B within 14 days after the diagnosis of pregnancy. Requires an approved laboratory report all positive or reactive tests. Requires all laboratory reports, files and records to be confidential and be opened only by authorized health officers or by written consent of the woman.

KS   **Kan. Stat. Ann § 65-153g (1992)** requires a physician or others required to report births and stillbirths to state on a separate sheet accompanying the birth or stillbirth certificate whether a blood test for syphilis was made during the pregnancy and the date for the test. Requires stating the reasons when a test is not completed.

Prohibits anything on the actual certificate that states whether the test was or was not made or the results of the tests.

KY   **Ky. Rev. Stat. § 214.170 (1995)** requires physician to identify on the sample as being from a pregnant woman when submitting it for syphilis test. Requires the laboratory to report any positive test result within one week after the examination.

LA   **La. Rev. Stat. Ann § 1093 (1992)** requires a physician and others required to make the reports to state on the birth or stillbirth certificate that a standard test for syphilis was completed.

ME   **Me. Rev. Stat. Ann. tit. 22, § 1232 (1992)** authorizes the department to approve one or more tests for syphilis. Allows the department to approve and appoint other laboratories in addition to the state laboratory to make a syphilis test. Requires that, with every positive syphilis test, the name, address, age and sex of the person be reported to the department.

MO   **Mo. Ann. Stat. § 210.040 (Vernon 1996)** requires reporting any positive syphilis or Hepatitis B tests to the department. Requires the report to be held confidential.

MO   **Mo. Ann. Stat. § 210.050 (Vernon 1996)** requires reporting on the birth or stillbirth certificate that blood tests for syphilis and Hepatitis B were made and the date of the tests. Prohibits stating the test results on a certificate.

MO   **Mo. Ann. Stat. § 210.060 (Vernon 1996)** makes it a misdemeanor for any licensed physician, midwife, registered nurse or other person who provides health care to a pregnant woman and who misrepresents the facts required for reporting any positive blood tests for syphilis or Hepatitis B. Requires that the crime be punishable by imprisonment of no more than a year, or by a fine of no more than $1,000, or both.

NE   **Neb. Rev. Stat. § 71-502.03 (1996)** requires a physician to take a blood sample of a pregnant woman at the time of the first examination and submit it for a standard serological test for syphilis to an approved laboratory. Requires the results be reported to the state. Requires a fee to cover the cost of the test. Requires a physician to report on the birth or stillbirth certificate that a blood test for syphilis was completed on the mother and the approximate date of the test. Prohibits stating the test results on a certificate. Requires the reason to be stated if the test was not performed.

NJ   **N.J. Stat. Ann. § 26:4-49.3 (West 1996)** requires a physician or other person to make reports to the state on the birth or stillbirth certificate that a blood test for syphilis was completed and the approximate date of the test.

OH   **Ohio Rev. Code Ann. § 3701.46 (Page 1997)** requires a physician or other required medical personnel to report on the birth or fetal death certificate that blood tests for syphilis and gonorrhea were performed on the mother and approximate dates of the tests. Prohibits stating the test results on the birth or fetal death certificate.

OH   **Ohio Rev. Code Ann. § 3701.48 (Page 1997)** requires a laboratory making the standard tests for syphilis and gonorrhea to give a report to the physician or health commissioner submitting the specimens. Requires laboratories to report any reactive syphilis test or positive gonorrhea test to the department.

OK   **Okla. Stat. Ann. tit. 43, § 33 (1990)** outlines the procedure for reporting results of a premarital test for syphilis by the doctor and laboratory. Requires the doctor to file results with the state. Requires the results be confidential and not open to public inspection.

OK   **Okla. Stat. Ann. tit. 63, § 1-516 (1997)** requires a physician to report on a birth or stillbirth certificate whether a blood test for syphilis was made during the pregnancy. Requires the date of the test and the reason if the test was not given. Prohibits stating the test results on the certificate.

SD   **S.D. Codified Laws Ann. § 34-23-12 (1994)** requires a physician to report on the birth or stillbirth certificate that a blood test for syphilis was made and the approximate date of the test. Requires a reason be given when the test is not completed. Prohibits stating the test results on the birth certificate.

VT   **Vt. Stat. Ann. tit. 18, § 1092 (1982)** requires any physician or other qualified person providing medical care to a person infected with gonorrhea or syphilis to report the case to the state. Requires the infected person submit to treatment until discharged by a physician. Stipulates that any person who refuses treatment be reported to the state and punished by a fine of no more than $100, or three months in prison, or both.

VT   **Vt. Stat. Ann. tit. 18, § 1103 (1982)** requires the birth or stillbirth certificate to report whether a blood test for syphilis was done and the date of the test. Requires stating why a blood test was not completed. Prohibits stating the test results on the certificate.

WV   **W. Va. Code § 16-4-11 (1995)** requires a physician to report and to notify the local health officer of any person who is suspected of having syphilis, gonorrhea or chancroid and is exposing others to the infection. Requires the local health officer to investigate any suspected venereal disease cases.

WV   **W. Va. Code § 16-4-6 (1995)** requires any physician, hospital or penal institution to report a diagnosis or treatment of a syphilis, gonorrhea or chancroid case to the local municipal health officer and to the director of health.

WV   **W. Va. Code § 16-4A-3 (1995)** requires a physician to test the blood of a pregnant woman for syphilis and indicate on the blood sample that the blood specimen is from a pregnant woman. Outlines reporting requirements and requires the results be reported to the state. Requires all laboratory results and reports of a syphilis test for a pregnant woman be confidential and not be open for public inspection.

WV   **W. Va. Code § 16-4A-4 (1995)** requires reporting on the birth or stillbirth certificate that a blood test for syphilis was performed and the approximate date. Prohibits stating the test results on the birth or stillbirth certificate.

Sexual Assault/Offenders

AK   **Alaska Stat. § 18.15.300** allows the court to order a person charged with a sex offense to be tested for HIV or STDs. Allows an alleged victim, parent or guardian, or attorney to petition the court to order tests. Requires copies of the test results be provided to the charged sex offender, each requesting victim, or, if the victim is a minor, the parent or guardian.

AK   **Alaska Stat. § 18.15.310** requires that all blood drawn for a court-ordered HIV or STD test of a person charged with a sex offense be performed by a physician, physician's assistant or other qualified personnel and tested in a medically approved laboratory. Requires all test results that indicate exposure to or infection by HIV or other STDs be reported to the department. Requires anyone who receives test results, other than the test subjects, maintain confidentiality. Requires the department provide free counseling and free testing to the victim for HIV and other STDs, and counseling to the alleged sex offender upon request of the offender. Requires the department to provide referral to appropriate health care facilities and support services at the request of the victim.

AK   **Alaska Stat. § 18.15.320** requires the cost for testing a person charged with a sex offense for HIV and other STDs be paid by the department. Requires the court to order the person to pay for the tests if convicted of the sex offense charge.

CT   **Conn. Gen. Stat. § 54-102a (1997)** allows a court to order persons charged with certain sexual offenses to undergo a venereal examination and HIV testing. Requires reporting the results to the department. Allows the court to order treatment if HIV or a venereal disease is found. Requires the examination or test be paid for by the department. Makes it a Class C misdemeanor for any person who fails to comply with any court-ordered testing or treatment.

FL   **Fla. Stat. Ann. § 796.08 (West 1998)** requires a person already convicted of prostitution to be tested for HIV and STDs when arrested for prostitution. States the penalties for prostituting or soliciting another for prostitution while knowing of the infection and not informing the other person involved.

ID   **Idaho Code § 39-604 (Supplemental 1997)** requires testing and treating for a venereal disease and HIV for any person imprisoned in any state correctional facility. Requires testing and treating for a venereal disease for any person who is confined in any county or city jail when public health officials think there was exposure to an infection. Requires testing for HIV and Hepatitis B, any person, including a juvenile, who is charged with a sex offense or prostitution. Requires the court to release the test results to the victim or to the parent or guardian when the victim is a minor. Requires a prisoner to be entitled to HIV counseling when tested HIV positive and to receive referrals to appropriate health care and support services. Requires the victim to receive counseling and to receive referral services at the time of the test results.

IL   **Ill. Ann. Stat. ch. 410 § 70/5 (Smith-Hurd 1997)** requires minimum requirements for hospitals that provide emergency services to sexual assault survivors. Hospitals must offer sexual assault survivors a blood test to determine the presence of an STD, written and oral instructions indicating the need for a second blood test six weeks after the sexual assault to determine the presence or absence of an STD, appropriate oral and written information about the possibility of infection of an STD and pregnancy resulting from the sexual assault, oral and written information about accepted medical procedures and medication available for the prevention or treatment of a venereal disease infection resulting from a sexual assault, and information to provide or refer the victim to counseling.

KY   **Ky. Rev. Stat. § 529.090 (1996)** makes it a Class A misdemeanor for any person who commits prostitution when he or she tested positive for an STD and could possibly infect another person through sexual activity.

LA   **La. Rev. Stat. Ann § 15:535 (West 1992 and Supplemental)** authorizes the court to order an adjudicated delinquent or a person convicted of a sexual offense to submit to an STD or HIV test. Requires the procedure or test to be performed by a qualified physician who is required to report any positive result to the Department of Public Safety and Corrections. Requires notification of the test results to the victim or the parent, regardless of the results.

MN   **Minn. Stat. § 611A.20 (1996)** requires a hospital to give written information about STDs to a person receiving medical services who reports or shows evidence of sexual assault or unwanted sexual contact. Requires the contents to inform the victim of the risk of contracting STDs as a result of a sexual assault, the symptoms of STDs, recommendations for periodic testing for STDs, where confidential testing is done, and information necessary to make an informed decision about whether to request a test of the offender.

MS   **Miss. Code Ann. § 99-37-25 (Supplement 1997)** requires the county pay for the STD tests and medical examination of an alleged sex offender. Requires the test results be made available to the victim or to the parent or guardian of the victim if the victim is a child. Requires any defendant who is convicted of rape, sexual battery of a child, touching or handling of a child or exploiting a child pay the county for the STD tests and medical examination.

MT   **Mont. Code Ann. § 46-18-256 (1997)** outlines STD and HIV testing procedures for victims of sexual assault. Requires an offender to be tested for the presence of HIV or STDs at the request of the victim or the parent or guardian of the victim of a sexual offense. Requires the county attorney to release the test result to the convicted sexual offender and to the victim, or to the parent or guardian of the victim if the victim is a minor.

NV   **Nev. Rev. Stat. § 441A.320 (1993)** authorizes the health authority to test a person for STDs and HIV who is arrested for a sex offense crime. Requires the health authority to disclose the results to the victim or victim's parent or guardian if that person is a minor. Requires the health authority, at the request of the victim, provide an examination and counseling. Requires the court to order all expenses be paid by the offender.

NJ   **N.J. Stat. Ann. § 26:4-32 (West 1996)** requires a prostitute or other "lewd" person be considered a person suspected of being infected with a venereal disease and be required to submit to an examination at any time. Requires no certificate of freedom from a venereal disease be issued to any prostitute.

NM   **N. M. Stat. Ann. § 24-1-9.1 (1997)** allows for STD testing of persons convicted of certain criminal offenses. Allows the victim of a criminal sexual offense to petition the court to order a test be performed on the offender when a consent to perform a test cannot be obtained. Allows the parent or legal guardian to petition the court when the victim is a minor. Requires the court order to state that the test be administered to the offender within 10 days after the petition is filed. Requires the test results be disclosed only to the offender and the victim or the victim's parent or legal guardian.

NM   **N. M. Stat. Ann. § 24-1-9.2 (1997)** allows for STD testing of persons formally charged with or for allegedly committing certain criminal sexual offenses. Allows the victim of a criminal sexual offense to petition the court to order that a test be performed on the offender when consent to perform a test on an offender cannot be obtained, provided that the same test is first performed on the victim of the alleged criminal offense. Allows the parent or legal guardian to petition the court when the victim is a minor. Outlines court procedures. Requires court order to state that the offender be tested within 10 days after the petition is filed by the victim or parent. Allows results be disclosed only to the offender and the victim or the victim's parent or legal guardian. Allows for counseling for both the alleged offender and the victim.

NM   **N. M. Stat. Ann. § 24-1-9.6 (1997)** allows a victim of an alleged criminal offense who receives information about an STD test result to disclose the test results to protect the victim's health and safety, or the health and safety of the victim's family or sexual partner.

NM   **N. M. Stat. Ann. § 30-9-5 (1994)** allows the court to order a venereal disease examination and treatment for a person convicted of prostitution or soliciting a prostitute. Requires the state to pay for medical treatment when the infected person is unable to pay.

NY   **N.Y. Public Health Law § 2302 (McKinney 1993)** requires any person arrested for failure to comply with a court order for an STD examination, or arrested for frequenting houses of prostitution be examined for STDs. Outlines court procedures. Prohibits the release of any person convicted until that person has been examined.

NC   **N.C. Gen. Stat. § 15A-615 (1997)** allows testing a sex offender who has had an alleged sexual contact with any minor under age 16 for STDs including chlamydia, gonorrhea, Hepatitis B, herpes, HIV and syphilis. Allows the victim to petition the court for the offender to be tested. Requires the test results be reported to the local health director. Requires the victim and alleged offender be informed of the test results and be provided with counseling. Requires the results of the test not be admissible as evidence in any criminal proceeding.

ND   **N.D. Cent. Code § 23-07.7-01 (1997)** allows the court to order any defendant or any alleged juvenile offender charged with a sex offense to submit to medical testing for STDs. Allows the court to order the testing only if the court receives a petition from the alleged victim. Requires a copy of the test results be released to the defendant's or alleged juvenile offender's physician and each requesting victim's physician. Outlines court procedures.

ND   **N.D. Cent. Code § 23-07.7-02 (1997)** outlines testing procedures for court-ordered testing. Requires testing for HIV and STDs. Requires laboratory to send a copy of test results to the physician who supplies results to defendant and victim, and the department. Makes it a Class C felony for any person who violates confidentiality.

OH   **Ohio Rev. Code Ann. § 2907.27 (Page 1996)** requires any person charged with rape, sexual battery, corruption of a minor, solicitation, solicitation after being found HIV-positive, prostitution and prostitution after being found HIV-positive, to be tested for a venereal disease upon request of the victim. Requires the accused to submit to medical treatment if found to be suffering from a venereal disease in an infectious stage. Requires the cost of the medical treatment be paid by the accused. Requires the court to order the accused to report for treatment at a health facility operated by the city if the accused is unable to pay.

OK   **Okla. Stat. Ann. tit. 63, § 1-524 (1997)** requires examining all prisoners to determine if a prisoner is infected with an STD. Allows a licensed physician to examine persons who are arrested for prostitution or other sex crimes. Allows a person to be detained until the results are known. Requires any person found to be infected with an STD to be treated. Requires quarantining any person who refuses treatment. Requires a person who is arrested for rape and other serious sexual crimes be tested for STDs and HIV. Authorizes the court to issue an order for testing during the arraignment. Requires the order not to include the name and address of the alleged victim. Requires the alleged victim be notified of the test results.

OK   **Okla. Stat. Ann. tit. 63, § 1-525 (1997)** requires all information including the records and test results of an infected person charged with a sex offense, be confidential and be disclosed only by court order. Allows the victim of the crime to request the results of the examination and test results conducted on the offender. Requires the department to provide free testing to the alleged victim for any venereal or communicable disease when the offender tests positive for any tests. Requires that the testing of the victim be accompanied with pre-test and post-test counseling. Requires the state board of health to rule and regulate procedural guidelines for testing sex offenders and releasing records containing the sex offender's test results. Requires the guidelines to respect the rights of the person arrested for the alleged sex offense and the victim of the alleged sex offense.

PA   **Pa. Cons. Stat. Ann. tit. 35, § 521.8 (Purdon 1993)** allows any person taken into custody and charged with a sex offense crime to be examined for a venereal disease by a department or court-appointed physician. Allows any person convicted of a crime and suspected of being infected to be examined for a venereal disease. Requires treating any person found to be infected with a venereal disease.

PR   **P.R. Laws Ann. tit. 24, § 575a (1993)** mandates that all test results remain confidential except in minimal cases where the offender is confirmed HIV positive.

PR   **P.R. Laws Ann. tit. 24, § 578 (1993)** requires providers to work in coordination with the victim's assistance center when they find out that the sex offender is HIV positive.

SC   **S.C. Code Ann. § 16-15-255 (Law. Co-op 1997)** requires testing of certain sex offenders for Hepatitis B, STDs and HIV. Outlines court procedures. Requires the convicted offender to pay for the test unless the offender is indigent, then the tests will be paid for by the state. Requires the state provide the victim and the convicted offender with counseling if any of the tests are positive.

SC   **S.C. Code Ann. § 16-3-740 (Law. Co-op 1997)** requires testing of certain convicted offenders for Hepatitis B, STDs and HIV within 15 days of the conviction. Outlines court procedures. Requires the convicted offender or adjudicated juvenile offender to pay for the test unless the offender is indigent, then the tests will be paid for by the state. Requires the state to provide the victim and the convicted offender with counseling if any of the tests are positive.

TX   **Tex. Family Code Ann § 54.033 (Vernon 1996)** outlines juvenile justice proceedings for STD and HIV testing. Requires a juvenile found delinquent of certain crimes to undergo an STD and HIV/AIDS test at the direction of the court or at the request of the victim. Allows the court to order a test if the child refuses to consent to the procedure or test. Prohibits the court from releasing the test result to anyone other than an authorized person.

VT   **Vt. Stat. Ann. tit. 13, § 2634 (1974)** requires medical treatment given to a person convicted of prostitution and infected with a venereal disease before probation or parole be given to prevent the spread of such disease.

VA   **Va. Code § 32.1-36 (1997)** requires a physician who diagnoses a venereal disease in a child age 12 or younger to report the case to the authorities, unless the physician reasonably believes that the infection was acquired congenitally or by means other than sexual abuse. Requires all information reported be confidential.

VA   **Va. Code § 32.1-58 (1997)** requires a person convicted of prostitution, soliciting a prostitute or certain sexual crimes be examined and tested for a venereal disease and treated if infected.

WA   **Wash. Rev. Code Ann. § 70.24.105 (Supplemental 1997)** prohibits any person to disclose or be compelled to disclose the identity of any person who has investigated, considered or requested a test or treatment for an STD. Allows for the exchange of medical information with certain authorized medical and social services personnel, law enforcement officers or by court order. Allows disclosure of test results upon the request of a victim of a sex crime.

WV   **W. Va. Code § 16-4-5 (1995)** requires testing and treating any person who has been convicted of a sexual offense or sexual immorality. Requires not releasing any convicted person from custody until a local health officer has been notified and proper venereal disease tests have been given.

WI   **Wis. Stat. Ann. § 982.296 (West Supplement 1997)** requires testing a juvenile alleged of a sexual crime for HIV and other STDs. Allows the victim or alleged victim to request such order. Allows test results be disclosed to the parent or guardian of the juvenile, the victim or alleged victim, the parent or guardian if the victim or alleged victim is a child, the health care professional that provides care to the juvenile or the health care professional that provides care to the victim. Allows the court to order the county pay for the cost of the tests.

Testing—Gonorrhea/Chlamydia

AK   **Alaska Stat. § 18.15.270** requires the department to make available and use on a statewide basis the best current testing methods for detecting and diagnosing chlamydia and gonorrhea.

DE   **Del. Code Ann. tit. 16, § 708 (1996)** requires prenatal testing for syphilis, gonorrhea, chlamydia and other STDs during the first and second trimester of pregnancy and during delivery. Requires that specimens be taken by a qualified health care professional and submitted to an approved laboratory free of charge. Exempts testing for religious reasons.

NJ   **N.J. Stat. Ann. § 26:4-49.6 (West 1996)** requires a migrant laborer to submit to a syphilis, gonorrhea and venereal disease examination within 30 days after entering New Jersey to work, unless the migrant laborer can prove that a venereal disease was completed within the last 90 days. Requires any person who employs a migrant laborer to notify the state department of health within five days of the beginning of employment whether the person has been examined for a venereal disease.

NC   **N.C. Gen. Stat. § 15A-615 (1997)** allows testing a sex offender who has had an alleged sexual contact with any minor under age 16 for STDs including chlamydia, gonorrhea, Hepatitis B, herpes, HIV and syphilis. Allows the victim to petition the court for the offender to be tested. Requires the test results be reported to the local health director. Requires the victim and alleged offender be informed of the test results and be provided with counseling. Requires the results of the test not be admissible as evidence in any criminal proceeding.

OH   **Ohio Rev. Code Ann. § 3701.47 (Page 1997)** requires that the standard tests for syphilis and gonorrhea be tests approved by the department. Requires all standard tests be made in an approved laboratory. Requires tests be made without charge when requested by a physician.

OH   **Ohio Rev. Code Ann. § 3701.49 (Page 1997)** requires that a person who is allowed to attend a pregnant woman but who is not authorized to take a blood sample notify the health commissioner of the case. Requires the health commissioner to take a test specimen of the pregnant woman and submit it for a standard syphilis and gonorrhea test.

OH   **Ohio Rev. Code Ann. § 3701.50 (Page 1997)** requires a physician to take a blood specimen of a pregnant woman within 10 days of the first examination and submit it to an approved laboratory for standard syphilis and gonorrhea tests. Requires a specimen be taken soon after delivery if a specimen cannot be taken prior to the delivery. Allows for religious exemption with written proof that the tests required are contrary to the practices of the religious belief.

Testing—Other

AL   **Ala. Code § 22-11A-13 (1997)** authorizes and directs the Board of Health to declare rules for testing, reporting, investigation and treatment of STDs.

AL   **Ala. Code § 22-11A-23 (1997)** requires any person who the state or county health officer has reason to believe has been exposed to STDs to be tested. Requires any person who the state or county health officer has reason to believe is infected with STDs to seek and accept treatment at the direction of the health officer or a licensed physician.

CA   **Cal. Health & Safety Code § 120540 (West 1996)** allows the department to require a physician to test a patient infected or suspected of being infected with a venereal disease.

CA   **Cal. Health & Safety Code § 120545 (West 1996)** allows for an STD examination to be made at authorized laboratories.

CA   **Cal. Health & Safety Code § 120550 (West 1996)** allows for a person to receive additional venereal disease testing at other facilities.

CA   **Cal. Health & Safety Code § 120560 (West 1996)** requires an infected person be tested and examined periodically to determine the status of their STD.

CA   **Cal. Health & Safety Code § 120580 (West 1996)** authorizes a trained venereal disease case investigator employed by the health department who meets certain requirements to perform venipuncture or skin puncture for the purpose of withdrawing blood for an STD test.

CA   **Cal. Health & Safety Code § 120710 (West 1996)** mandates the department to accept specimens for testing due to questions of accuracy from the past test.

DE   **Del. Code Ann. tit. 16, § 702 (1996)** outlines the reporting procedures for STDs. Requires any physician who diagnoses or treats STDs to report to the state or county health officer. Requires any lab that conducts STD testing report all positive or reactive tests. Requires all reports and documentation be held confidential. Authorizes the state or county to follow appropriate procedures for infection control.

DE   **Del. Code Ann. tit. 16, § 705 (1996)** outlines emergency public health procedures for suspected or infected persons who refuse testing, examination or treatment and who present a threat to the public health. Allows the director of the Division of Public Health to ask the court for an injunction or to take the infected person into custody.

DE   **Del. Code Ann. tit. 16, § 708 (1996)** requires prenatal testing for syphilis, gonorrhea, chlamydia and other STDs during the first and second trimester of pregnancy and during delivery. Requires that specimens be taken by a qualified health care professional and submitted to an approved laboratory free of charge. Exempts testing for religious reasons.

DE   **Del. Code Ann. tit. 16, § 709 (1996)** authorizes trained STD case investigators to withdraw blood for test purposes even though he or she is not licensed to withdraw blood. Requires certain standards be met.

FL   **Fla. Stat. Ann. § 384.287 (West 1998)** allows for an officer, firefighter or paramedic who may have been exposed to an STD in the line of duty to request testing of the person they were exposed to as well as be tested themselves. Allows for a court order if the suspected person does not volunteer for testing. States that results are exempt from confidentiality.

HI   **Hawaii Rev. Stat. § 325-52 (1993)** outlines serologic testing and reporting. Requires requested tests to be free of charge when completed at a department laboratory. Requires the department to issue a "laboratory report form." Outlines the procedure for reporting.

ID   **Idaho Code § 39-601A (1993)** requires governmental authorities to provide services authorized or mandated by the law for treating or testing venereal diseases only to the extent of funding and available resources appropriate.

IL   **Ill. Ann. Stat. ch. 410 § 325/10 (Smith-Hurd 1997)** requires the department to adopt the rules necessary to perform the duties of the department. Requires rules of the department to include criteria, standards and procedures for the identification, investigation, examination and treatment of STDs.

IN   **Ind. Code Ann. § 16-41-14-1 (Burns 1993)** exempts testing of the semen of a donor for STDs when the donor is the husband of the recipient of artificial insemination.

IN   **Ind. Code Ann. § 16-41-14-6 (Burns 1993)** requires the department to adopt rules for STD testing of semen used in artificial insemination, including the identification of which diseases need to be tested and which type of test is to be used.

IA   **Iowa Code § 140.14 (1997)** allows for a religious exemption for the testing and treatment of a venereal disease.

LA   **La. Rev. Stat. Ann § 1067 (West 1992)** requires the secretary of the department to make rules and regulations for the diagnosis, treatment, reporting and prevention of venereal diseases.

MI   **Mich. Stat. Ann. § 14.15 (5119) (Law. Co-op 1995)** requires a marriage applicant be counseled by a physician or other authorized medical personnel on the transmission and prevention of venereal diseases and HIV infection. Requires a county clerk to distribute to each applicant educational materials prepared by the department about testing and counseling for a venereal diseases and HIV. Prohibits a county clerk from issuing a marriage license to an applicant who fails to present a certificate indicating the applicant has received counseling regarding the transmission and prevention of venereal diseases and HIV from a physician and has been offered or referred for venereal disease or HIV testing.

MI   **Mich. Stat. Ann. § 14.15 (5121) (Law. Co-op 1995)** makes it a misdemeanor for a county clerk to issue a marriage license to an individual who fails to present a certificate stating the applicant has received counseling about venereal diseases and HIV and has been offered venereal disease and HIV testing. Makes it a misdemeanor for any person who discloses the marriage license applicant has taken a venereal disease or HIV test and discloses the results of the tests except when required by law. Makes it a misdemeanor for a physician who knowingly and willfully makes a false statement in a certificate required for a marriage license.

MI   **Mich. Stat. Ann. § 14.15 (5123) (Law. Co-op 1995)** requires a physician to take blood samples of a pregnant woman and submit the specimens to an approved laboratory for HIV, Hepatitis B and venereal disease tests. Requires testing the woman at the time of delivery if the tests have not already been completed. Allows for exemption if the tests are medically inadvisable or the woman refuses to be tested.

MN   **Minn. Stat. § 62Q.14 (1996)** prohibits any health insurance plan to restrict the choice of an enrollee as to where the enrollee receives services related to testing and treatment of STDs.

MS   **Miss. Code Ann. § 41-23-30 (1993)** requires the county health departments to provide free testing and treatment for STDs. Requires all testing and treatment be held confidential. Requires using available media to advertise the confidentiality of the test and treatment.

MT   **Mont. Code Ann. § 50-19-107 (1997)** requires laboratory results of an STD test be shown by the physician to the patient. Allows the report of the results to be shown, upon request of the patient, to the spouse of the patient or, if the patient is a minor, to the minor's parents or the minor's legal guardian.

NJ   **N.J. Stat. Ann. § 26:4-47 (West 1996)** allows free diagnosis and treatment of STDs to be provided by the state Department of Health. Allows the commissioner of health to establish rules and regulations pertaining to the payment for services and educational materials provided by the department.

NY   **N.Y. Public Health Law § 2304 (McKinney 1993)** requires that the Board of Health provide adequate facilities for the free diagnosis and treatment of persons suspected of being infected or who are infected with an STD. Authorizes the health officer to administer these facilities. Allows a person to be treated at his own expense by a licensed physician of his choice. Requires facilities to comply with the requirements of the commissioner.

NY   **N.Y. Public Health Law § 2305 (McKinney 1993)** prohibits any person other than a licensed physician from diagnosing, treating or prescribing medicine to a person infected with an STD. Allows a licensed physician to diagnose, treat or prescribe for a person under age 21without the consent or knowledge of a parent or guardian.

NY   **N.Y. Public Health Law § 2308-a (McKinney 1993)** requires the administrative officer or other person in charge of a health clinic providing medical treatment for women to offer every resident coming to such clinics or facilities for treatment, appropriate examinations or tests for the detection of STDs.

NY   **N.Y. Public Health Law § 2309 (McKinney 1993)** makes it a misdemeanor for any person who violates the rules and regulations of the department regarding testing, reporting and confidentiality of STDs.

ND **N.D. Cent. Code § 23-07-07 (1991)** authorizes the state, local and city health officers, when necessary for the protection of public health, to examine any person suspected of being infected with an STD, to require any person to report for treatment, to investigate any cases and to cooperate with other officials to enforce the laws.

PA **Pa. Cons. Stat. Ann. tit. 35, 521.9 (Purdon 1993)** requires the department to provide free diagnosis and treatment for anyone with a venereal disease. Allows any local board or department to share in the financial support for providing free diagnosis and treatment for a venereal disease.

PA **Pa. Cons. Stat. Ann. tit. 35,521.14 (Purdon 1993)** requires all STD tests be approved by the department. Requires all tests be made in a department-approved laboratory.

PR **P.R. Laws Ann. tit. 24, § 576 (1993)** requires health workers to advise an individual to be tested for an STD when they suspect the person may be infectious to others.

PR **P.R. Laws Ann. tit. 24, § 577 (1993)** states that it is a provider's responsibility to test minors and developmentally disabled people for STDs.

RI **R.I. Gen. Laws § 23-11-4 (1996)** authorizes the department to establish a reasonable fee structure for state laboratory tests and clinical treatments.

RI **R.I. Gen. Laws § 23-11-12 (1996)** makes it a misdemeanor for any person who refuses an examination for STDs and, upon conviction, be punished a $50 fine, or by imprisonment for 30 days, or both.

VT **Vt. Stat. Ann. tit. 18, § 1094 (1982)** allows any person suspected of being infected with a venereal disease to petition the court so that no examination or tests be made. Requires the petition not be a public record. Requires the suspected person be informed of the right to petition.

VT **Vt. Stat. Ann. tit. 18, § 1098 (1982)** requires the board to provide free testing for suspected venereal disease cases and provide free hospitalization and other treatment for infected patients who are unable to pay. Requires the board not to pay for the diagnosis and treatment until all required reports are completed by the physician and supplied to the board.

VA **Va. Code § 32.1-56 (1997)** requires a physician or any other person who examines or treats a person having a venereal disease to provide information to the infected person about the disease, the nature of the disease, methods of treatment, prevention of the spread of the disease, and the necessity of tests to ensure that a cure has been accomplished.

VA **Va. Code § 32.1-59 (1997)** requires any person admitted to any state correctional institution or state hospital to be examined and tested for a venereal disease. Requires the institution to provide treatment and report the case.

WA **Wash. Rev. Code Ann. § 70.24.050 (1996)** requires that a diagnosis of an STD be confirmed by a test from an approved laboratory.

WA **Wash. Rev. Code Ann. § 70.24.120 (1996)** authorizes STD case investigators to perform venipuncture or skin puncture on a person for an STD test. Requires the investigator be trained and possess a statement signed by the training physician.

WV **W. Va. Code § 16-4-19 (1995)** allows a person to voluntarily submit to an examination and treatment for a venereal disease. Allows the person to receive treatment at a local clinic free of charge if that person is unable to pay.

WI **Wis. Stat. Ann. § 252.10 (West Supplemental 1997)** requires state laboratories to examine specimens for any physician or local health officer in the state for the diagnosis of STDs. Requires all laboratories to report all positive results to the local health officer and to the department with the name of the physician who diagnosed the case.

WI **Wis. Stat. Ann. § 252.10 (West Supplemental 1997)** requires programs in counties with an incidence of gonorrhea, chlamydia or syphilis that exceeds the statewide average, to diagnose and treat STDs at no cost to the patient. Requires the county board of supervisors to be responsible for ensuring that the program exists, but boards are required to establish their own programs only if no other public or private program is operating. Requires the department to compile statistics indicating the incidence of gonorrhea, chlamydia and syphilis for each county in the state.

WI   **Wis. Stat. Ann. § 252.10 (West Supplemental 1997)** allows a health care professional to test an individual for STDs without first obtaining informed consent to do the testing. Prohibits disclosure of name of test subject on any sample used for performance of an STD test.

WY   **Wyo. Stat. § 35-4-130 (1997)** makes it a misdemeanor for any person violating or refusing to comply with the rules and regulations regarding STD testing, treatment and reporting, and is punishable by a fine of no more than $750, imprisonment for no more than six months, or both.

WY   **Wyo. Stat. § 35-4-131 (1997)** allows a person under age 18 to give legal consent for the examination and treatment of any STD infection. Requires a physician, health officer, or other person or facility providing health care to administer treatment or refer appropriate treatment of any person reasonably suspected of being infected or exposed to an STD. States that a physical examination and treatment of a consenting person under age 18 by a licensed physician or other qualified health care provider is not an assault on that person.

WY   **Wyo. Stat. § 35-4-133 (1997)** allows a health worker to request testing of a possibly STD-infected person. Allows the county to apply for a court order to have a test performed if the patient does not consent to testing. Requires test results be kept confidential and reported to the state.

Testing—Pregnant Women and Newborns

AL   **Ala. Code § 22-11A-16 (1997)** establishes the procedure for serologic syphilis testing for pregnant women during the first and third trimesters. Requires the samples be submitted to an approved laboratory. Requires testing newborns for syphilis. Requires reporting all positive or reactive tests.

AK   **Alaska Stat. § 18.15.150** defines prenatal testing protocol for syphilis. Requires a blood sample be taken at the first professional visit or within 10 days after the visit and submitted to an approved laboratory. Allows for religious exemption.

AK   **Alaska Stat. § 18.15.170** requires a report on the birth or death certificate to state whether the woman who bore the child had been tested for syphilis. Prohibits stating test results on the birth or death certificate.

AK   **Alaska Stat. § 18.15.180** requires a physician to take a blood sample from a pregnant woman for syphilis. Makes it a misdemeanor for any physician who does not take a blood sample for syphilis, punishable by a fine of a maximum of $500. Exempts physicians whose patient refused testing.

AZ   **Ariz. Rev. Stat. Ann. § 36-693 (1993)** requires a physician to take a blood sample of a pregnant woman at the first prenatal exam and submit it to an approved laboratory for a standard serological syphilis test. Requires that a blood sample from the umbilical cord be taken at the delivery if the mother did not have a syphilis test prior to the delivery. Requires the test be free of charge.

AZ   **Ariz. Rev. Stat. Ann. § 36-694 (1993)** requires a physician to report on the birth or stillbirth certificate that a blood test for syphilis was made either from the mother or from the umbilical cord at the delivery and the approximate date when the specimen was taken.

AR   **Ark. Stat. Ann. § 20-16-507 (1991)** requires a physician to take a blood sample of a pregnant woman and submit the sample to an approved laboratory for a standard serological test for syphilis. Requires others not allowed by law to take blood but allowed to attend a pregnant woman, to make sure the procedure is completed. Requires tests be free of charge when requested. Requires a physician and others authorized to make reports, to state on the birth or stillbirth certificate that a blood sample was taken for a syphilis test and the approximate date.

CA   **Cal. Health & Safety Code § 120685 (West 1996)** requires a physician or other prenatal care provider to submit a blood sample from the pregnant woman for syphilis at the first professional visit or within 10 days of the first visit or at the time of delivery.

CA   **Cal. Health & Safety Code § 120690 (West 1996)** requires the blood sample of a pregnant woman be submitted to an approved laboratory for a standard syphilis test.

CA   **Cal. Health & Safety Code § 120695 (West 1996)** requires a physician, when testing for syphilis, to designate the sample submitted to the laboratory as a prenatal test or a test following delivery.

CA   **Cal. Health & Safety Code § 120715 (West 1996)** makes it a misdemeanor for any licensed physician or surgeon attending a pregnant or recently delivered woman to not obtain a blood sample for syphilis. Stipulates the authorized person is not guilty if the test is refused by the patient.

CA   **Cal. Health & Safety Code § 125085 (West 1996)** requires a blood specimen of a pregnant woman be submitted to an approved public health lab to determine the presence of Hepatitis B. Requires the test results be reported to the attending physician and the woman tested.

CA   **Cal. Health & Safety Code § 125100 (West 1996)** requires prenatal care providers and laboratories to provide the department with information necessary to evaluate the effectiveness of testing and follow-up treatment for the prevention of perinatally transmitted Hepatitis B. Mandates the department to make available, depending on funding, money to counties who request funding for testing and follow-up treatment for preventing perinatally transmitted Hepatitis B infection.

CO   **Colo. Rev. Stat. § 25-4-201 (1990)** requires a physician to take a blood sample of a pregnant woman within 10 days of the first professional visit and submit it to an approved laboratory for a standard serological test for syphilis.

CO	**Colo. Rev. Stat. § 25-4-202 (1997)** requires the standard prenatal serological test for syphilis be approved by the department and conducted at laboratories approved by the department. Allows for tests to be free of charge.
CO	**Colo. Rev. Stat. § 25-4-203 (1990)** requires a physician to report on the birth or stillbirth certificate that a blood test for syphilis was conducted the approximate date of the test. Prohibits stating the test result on the birth certificate.
CO	**Colo. Rev. Stat. § 25-4-204 (1990)** makes it a misdemeanor, with a fine of no more than $300, for any physician to not take a blood sample from a pregnant woman and submit it for a syphilis test. Releases any physician whose patient refuses to give a syphilis test from being found guilty of a misdemeanor.
CT	**Conn. Gen. Stat. § 19a-90 (1997)** establishes the procedure for testing all pregnant women for syphilis. Requires a physician to take a blood sample from a pregnant woman within 30 days from the date of the first examination and during the final trimester. Requires tests be submitted to an approved laboratory for a standard serological test. Requires testing be made free of charge.
DE	**Del. Code Ann. tit. 16, § 708 (1996)** requires prenatal testing for syphilis, gonorrhea, chlamydia and other STDs during the first and second trimester of pregnancy and during delivery. Requires that specimens be taken by a qualified health care professional and submitted to an approved laboratory free of charge. Exempts testing for religious reasons.
FL	**Fla. Stat. Ann. § 384.31 (West 1998)** requires the serological testing of pregnant women for STDs and HIV.
HI	**Hawaii Rev. Stat. § 325-51 (1993)** requires a pregnant woman be tested for syphilis and the test be submitted to an approved laboratory. Requires samples be taken during the period of gestation adopted by the department.
HI	**Hawaii Rev. Stat. § 325-53 (1993)** requires a report accompany the birth or death certificate that states a woman who gave birth to a child was tested for syphilis. States that failure to test or report for syphilis may be punishable up to a $1,000 fine per violation.
ID	**Idaho Code § 39-1001 (1993)** requires a physician attending a pregnant woman to take a serological syphilis test within 15 days of the first examination and at the time of delivery. Requires the physician to specify whether it was a prenatal test or a test following recent delivery when submitting to the laboratory. Allows a fee to be collected.
ID	**Idaho Code § 39-1002 (1993)** requires a person attending a pregnant or recently delivered woman who is not a licensed physician and is not permitted to take blood samples to ensure that the syphilis testing procedure is completed by a licensed physician and an approved laboratory.
ID	**Idaho Code § 39-1005 (1993)** requires a report on the birth certificate to state whether the woman who bore the child has been tested for syphilis. Prohibits stating the test result on the birth or death certificate.
ID	**Idaho Code § 39-1006 (1993)** states that any authorized medical person who does not request a syphilis test on a pregnant woman or a woman who recently delivered be found guilty of a misdemeanor. Stipulates that, if testing is refused by the patient, the authorized person requesting the test be found not guilty of a misdemeanor.
IL	**Ill. Ann. Stat. ch. 410 § 320/1 (Smith-Hurd 1997)** requires serological testing of pregnant women for syphilis during the first examination and during the third trimester. Requires all tests be submitted to an approved laboratory. Requires additional testing with a positive or doubtful test result. Requires any test requested by a physician to be free of charge. Allows for religious exemption.
IL	**Ill. Ann. Stat. ch. 410 § 320/2 (Smith-Hurd 1997)** requires a birth or death certificate to state whether the woman who bore the child has been tested for syphilis. Prohibits giving the test results on the birth or death certificate.
IN	**Ind. Code Ann. § 16-41-15-10 (Burns 1997)** requires a physician take a blood sample from a pregnant woman at the time of first diagnosis and submit the sample to an approved laboratory for a standard serological test for syphilis. Requires a physician take a blood sample from a pregnant woman during the third trimester of pregnancy if the woman belongs to a high risk population recommended to test by the federal Centers for Disease Control--Sexually Transmitted Diseases Treatment Guidelines.

IN   **Ind. Code Ann. § 16-41-15-11 (Burns 1993)** requires an authorized person, who is permitted by law to attend a pregnant woman but who is not permitted by law to take blood specimens, ensure that a blood sample of a pregnant woman be taken by a licensed physician. Requires the sample be submitted to an approved laboratory for a standard serological test for syphilis.

IN   **Ind. Code Ann. § 16-41-15-12 (Burns 1993)** requires an authorized person take a blood sample of a woman, when at the time of delivery, evidence is not available to show that a standard serological test for syphilis has been made. Stipulates tgat samples must be submitted to an approved laboratory for a standard serological test for syphilis.

IN   **Ind. Code Ann. § 16-41-15-13 (Burns 1993)** outlines procedures required by the health department for reporting a serological test for syphilis on a birth or stillbirth certificate. Requires the date of the test and whether the test was made during pregnancy or at the time of delivery. Requires stating the reason if the test was not done.

IA   **Iowa Code § 140.11 (1997)** requires a physician or any other person required by law to attend a pregnant woman to take a blood sample for a syphilis test within 14 days of the first exam and submit it to an approved laboratory. Requires the husband or father of the child and the other children be given a blood test when the pregnant woman's syphilis test is positive.

IA   **Iowa Code § 140.12 (1997)** requires a physician to report on the birth or stillbirth certificate that a blood test for syphilis was made and the approximate date of the test. Requires reporting when the test is not given. Prohibits stating the test result on the birth certificate.

KS   **Kan. Stat. Ann § 65-153f (Supplemental 1997)** requires a physician or a person attending a pregnant woman, with the consent of the woman, to take a blood sample for a serological test for syphilis and Hepatitis B within 14 days after the diagnosis of pregnancy. Requires an approved laboratory report all positive or reactive tests. Requires all laboratory reports, files and records to be confidential and be opened only by authorized health officers or by written consent of the woman.

KY   **Ky. Rev. Stat. § 214.160 (1995)** requires a physician to take a blood sample from a pregnant woman or a suspected pregnancy and submit the sample to an approved laboratory for a serological test for syphilis. Requires a blood sample be taken within 10 days after delivery when the woman is in labor at the time of diagnosis of the pregnancy.

LA   **La. Rev. Stat. Ann § 1091 (West 1992)** requires a physician to take a blood sample at the time of a pregnant woman's first examination and submit the sample to an approved laboratory for a standard test for syphilis. Requires others permitted by law to attend a pregnant woman but not permitted to take a blood sample assure the sample is taken.

MA   **Mass. Gen. Laws Ann. ch. 111, § 121A (West 1996)** requires a physician attending a pregnant woman to take a blood sample during the first examination and submit the sample for a standard serological test for syphilis to a laboratory approved by the department.

ME   **Me. Rev. Stat. Ann. tit. 22, § 1231 (1992)** requires a physician to take a blood sample of a pregnant woman with her consent, and submit it to an approved laboratory for a standard serological syphilis test. Requires the test be free of charge.

MD   **Md. Health Code Ann. § 18-307 (1994)** requires testing pregnant women and infants for syphilis. Requires an authorized individual attending a pregnant woman to submit a blood sample to an approved medical laboratory. The sample should be drawn from the woman at the first examination and during the third trimester of pregnancy.

MI   **Mich. Stat. Ann. § 14.15 (5123) (Law. Co-op 1995)** requires a physician to take blood samples of a pregnant woman and submit the specimens to an approved laboratory for HIV, Hepatitis B and venereal disease tests. Requires testing the woman at the time of delivery if the tests have not already been completed. Allows for exemption if the tests are medically inadvisable or the woman refuses to be tested.

MO   **Mo. Ann. Stat. § 210.030 (Vernon 1996)** requires a physician or a qualified medical person to take a blood sample of a pregnant woman within 20 days of her first examination and submit it to an approved laboratory for a standard serological test for syphilis and Hepatitis B. Requires the test to be free of charge.

MT   **Mont. Code Ann. § 50-19-103 (1997)** requires every female, regardless of age or marital status, seeking prenatal care from a physician, to submit a blood specimen for a standard serological test for syphilis. Requires the physician or an authorized person who attends a pregnant woman take a blood sample at the first

112

professional visit and submit it to a laboratory. Requires the physician designate it as a prenatal test when submitting. Penalizes any physician or authorized person required to take the blood sample who violates this statute with a misdemeanor. Exempts any physician or authorized person who requests a sample and is refused by the patient.

MT   **Mont. Code Ann. § 50-19-110 (1997)** requires a birth or fetal death certificate to state whether a standard serological syphilis test was made, but prohibits stating the result of the test. Requires the certificate to state the approximate date when the specimen was taken and, if no test was made, the stated reason.

NE   **Neb. Rev. Stat. § 71-502.03 (1996)** requires a physician to take a blood sample of a pregnant woman at the time of the first examination and submit it for a standard serological test for syphilis at an approved laboratory. Requires the results be reported to the state. Requires a fee to cover the cost of the test. Requires a physician to report on the birth or stillbirth certificate that a blood test for syphilis was completed on the mother and the approximate date of the test. Prohibits stating the result of the test on a birth certificate. Requires the reason to be stated if the test was not performed.

NV   **Nev. Rev. Stat. § 442.010 (1993)** requires a physician or any authorized person to take a blood sample of a pregnant woman during the third trimester and submit it to a qualified laboratory for a standard serological test for syphilis. Requires that tests made in a state laboratory be free of charge. Allows for religious exemption.

NJ   **N.J. Stat. Ann. § 26:4-49.1 (West 1996)** requires a physician to take a blood sample of a pregnant woman at the first examination and submit it to an approved laboratory for a standard serological test for syphilis.

NJ   **N.J. Stat. Ann. § 26:4-49.3 (West 1996)** requires a physician or other person to make reports to the state on the birth or stillbirth certificate that a blood test for syphilis was completed and the approximate date of the test.

NM   **N. M. Stat. Ann. § 24-1-10 (1997)** requires a physician to take a blood sample of a pregnant woman at the first examination and submit the sample to the state public health laboratory for a standard serological test for syphilis. Requires tests be free of charge.

NM   **N. M. Stat. Ann. § 24-1-11 (1997)** requires a physician or other authorized person to state on the birth or stillbirth certificate whether a blood test for syphilis was made and approximate date when the specimen was taken.

NY   **N.Y. Public Health Law § 2308 (McKinney 1993)** requires a physician to take a blood sample of a pregnant women during the first examination and submit the sample to an approved laboratory for a standard serological test for syphilis.

OH   **Ohio Rev. Code Ann. § 3701.49 (Page 1997)** requires a person allowed to attend a pregnant woman but not authorized to take a blood sample to notify the health commissioner of the case. Requires the health commissioner to take a test specimen of the pregnant woman and submit it for standard syphilis and gonorrhea tests.

OH   **Ohio Rev. Code Ann. § 3701.50 (Page 1997)** requires a physician to take a blood specimen of the pregnant woman within 10 days of the first examination and submit it to an approved laboratory for standard syphilis and gonorrhea tests. Requires a specimen be taken soon after delivery if a specimen cannot be taken prior to the delivery. Allows for religious exemption with written proof that the tests required are contrary to the practices of the religious belief.

OK   **Okla. Stat. Ann. tit. 63, § 1-515 (1997)** requires testing pregnant women for syphilis. Requires a blood sample be taken from a pregnant woman during the first examination and submitted to an approved laboratory for a standard serological test for syphilis.

OK   **Okla. Stat. Ann. tit. 63, § 1-516.1 (1997)** allows for religious exemption when testing pregnant women for syphilis.

OR   **Or. Rev. Stat. § 433.017 (1995)** requires testing a pregnant woman for syphilis within 10 days of the first visit and requires the blood sample be submitted to an approved laboratory. Prohibits any sample from being taken without the pregnant woman's consent.

PA   **Pa. Cons. Stat. Ann. tit. 35, § 521.13 (Purdon 1993)** requires a physician to take a blood sample from a pregnant woman during the first examination or within 15 days of the first examination, and to submit the sample to an approved laboratory for a serological test for syphilis. Requires the physician to explain to the pregnant woman the usefulness of the test if she refuses. Requires the test be free of charge.

RI **R.I. Gen. Laws § 23-11-8 (1996)** requires a physician to obtain a blood specimen from a pregnant woman within 30 days after the first professional visit. Requires the blood specimen be submitted to the state laboratory or to an approved laboratory for a standard test for syphilis. Makes it a misdemeanor for failing to take a sample and requires a fine of no less than $10 and no more than $100.

SC **S.C. Code Ann. § 44-29-120 (Law. Co-op 1985)** requires a physician to take a blood sample of a pregnant woman within three days after her first examination and submit the sample to an approved laboratory for a standard serological test for syphilis, rubella and Rh factor. Requires other persons who are allowed to attend a pregnant woman but who are not allowed to take a blood sample, to ensure the sample is taken. Makes it a misdemeanor, punishable by a fine of no more than $100 and imprisonment for no more than 30 days, for anyone who does not take a sample for a syphilis test. Allows for religious exemption.

SD **S.D. Codified Laws Ann. § 34-23-9 (1994)** requires a physician to take a blood sample of a pregnant woman during her first examination and submit the sample to an approved laboratory for a standard serological test for syphilis.

SD **S.D. Codified Laws Ann. § 34-23-10 (1994)** requires a person who is not permitted by law to take a blood sample but who is authorized to attend a pregnant woman to make sure a blood sample is taken by a licensed physician and a syphilis test is completed.

SD **S.D. Codified Laws Ann. § 34-23-12 (1994)** requires a physician to report on the birth or stillbirth certificate that a blood test for syphilis was made and the approximate date of the test. Requires a reason be given when the test is not completed. Prohibits stating the test result the birth certificate.

TX **Tex. Health & Safety Code Ann. § 81.090 (Vernon 1992)** requires a physician to take a blood sample of a pregnant woman at the first examination and within 24 hours of the delivery and submit the sample to a certified laboratory for standard serological tests for syphilis and HIV. Outlines other duties required during the first exam, including distributing information about HIV/AIDS and syphilis, verbally notifying the woman that an HIV test will be performed, and advising the woman that the result of the test is not anonymous, and explaining the difference between an anonymous and confidential test. Prohibits the physician from conducting the HIV test if the woman objects to the test. Requires the physician to refer the woman to an anonymous testing site or instruct the woman about anonymous testing methods, if she objects to testing.

UT **Utah Code Ann. § 26-6-20 (1995)** requires a licensed physician or surgeon to take a blood sample of a pregnant woman within 10 days of her first examination and to submit the sample to an approved laboratory for a standard serological test for syphilis. Allows for religious exemption. Requires a copy of the results be given to the physician and a copy submitted to the department. Requires the test results be kept confidential and not open to public inspection.

VT **Vt. Stat. Ann. tit. 18, § 1102 (1982)** requires any authorized medical person to take a blood sample of a pregnant woman prior to the third month of pregnancy and submit the sample to an approved laboratory for a standard serological test for syphilis.

VA **Va. Code § 32.1-60 (1997)** requires any person attending a pregnant woman to take prenatal tests for venereal diseases within 15 days of the first examination. Requires the tests for venereal diseases be submitted to an approved laboratory.

VA **Va. Code § 32.1-73 (1997)** makes it punishable, with the penalty of losing their license, for physicians, nurses or midwives who fail to comply with testing a pregnant woman for venereal diseases.

WA **Wash. Rev. Code Ann. § 70.24.090 (1996)** requires a physician to take a blood sample of a pregnant woman during her first examination and submit the sample to an approved laboratory for a standard serological test for syphilis. Requires the physician to urge the patient to have the test before the fifth month of any following pregnancies if the first exam is after her fifth month.

WA **Wash. Rev. Code Ann. § 70.24.095 (1996)** requires a health care practitioner attending a pregnant woman or attending a drug treatment program participant who is seeking treatment of an STD to ensure that the patient receives AIDS counseling.

WV **W. Va. Code § 16-4A-1 (1995)** requires every pregnant woman to have a blood sample taken and submitted to an approved laboratory for a standard serologic test for syphilis.

WV **W. Va. Code § 16-4A-2 (1995)** requires a blood sample for a syphilis test be taken within 10 days of delivery if a specimen is not taken during the woman's pregnancy. Requires tests to be performed without charge.

114

WY **Wyo. Stat. § 35-4-501 (1997)** requires all standard serological tests for syphilis for pregnant women be performed at an approved laboratory and allows tests be performed without charge.

WY **Wyo. Stat. § 35-4-502 (1997)** requires a physician to take a blood sample of a pregnant woman within 10 days of her first professional visit and submit the sample to an approved laboratory for a standard serological test for syphilis.

WY **Wyo. Stat. § 35-4-503 (1997)** requires reporting on the birth or stillbirth certificate that a syphilis test was completed and the approximate date of the test. Prohibits stating the test results.

Testing—Prisoners

AL   **Ala. Code § 22-11A-17 (1997)** outlines STD testing and treatment procedures for correctional facility inmates. Requires testing of correctional facility inmates who are sentenced or confined for 30 or more consecutive days. States that inmates confined for more than 90 days are to be tested 30 days prior to release. Requires discharged infectious inmates be reported to the county or state health officers.

CO   **Colo. Rev. Stat. § 25-4-405 (1997)** requires any person confined, detained or imprisoned in any state or county hospital for the insane, mental institution, home for dependent children, reformatory, prison, or any private or charitable institution be examined and treated for a venereal disease. Requires a manager to make room available to the health authorities for quarantining and treating the confined person for a venereal disease. Requires any person infected with a venereal disease at the time of their release to be quarantined and treated at public expense. Authorizes the department to arrange for hospitalization.

CT   **Conn. Gen. Stat. § 18-94 (1997)** allows keeping a prison inmate who is infected with a venereal disease in the correctional or charitable institution longer than the date of the prisoner's discharge when the institution considers the inmate to be dangerous to the public health.

DE   **Del. Code Ann. tit. 16, § 706 (1996)** establishes protocol for the examination and treatment of prisoners. Requires reporting suspected, untreated prisoners upon release to a local health officer. Requires prison medical staff to adhere to current STD medical protocol. Requires the prison to inform the Division of Public Health when a person infected with or suspected of having an STD is released from prison without appropriate treatment, counseling or examination. Allows the division to examine medical records or other medical information to ensure that appropriate STD medical practices are followed. Requires all state, county and city prisons to provide space necessary to quarantine any person known or suspected of having an STD.

FL   **Fla. Stat. Ann. § 384.32 (West 1993)** authorizes the department to enter any state, county or municipal correctional facility to interview, examine or treat any prisoner suspected of being infected with STDs. Requires correctional facilities to cooperate.

ID   **Idaho Code § 39-604 (Supplemental 1997)** requires testing and treating for a venereal disease and HIV, any person imprisoned in any state correctional facility. Requires testing and treating for a venereal disease, any person confined in any county or city jail when public health officials think there was exposure to an infection. Requires testing any person, including a juvenile, for HIV and Hepatitis B when charged with a sex offense or prostitution. Requires the court to release the test results to the victim or to the parent or guardian when the victim is a minor. Requires a prisoner to be entitled to HIV counseling when tested HIV-positive and to receive referrals to appropriate health care and support services. Requires the victim to receive counseling and referral services at the time of the test results.

IL   **Ill. Ann. Stat. ch. 410 § 325/9 (Smith-Hurd 1997)** authorizes the department to interview, examine and treat any prisoner for an STD. Requires any state, county or municipal detention facility to cooperate.

IN   **Ind. Code Ann. § 16-4-15-16 (Burns 1993)** requires the state laboratory to provide venereal disease tests free of charge to diagnose and test a prisoner.

IN   **Ind. Code Ann. § 16-41-15-15 (Burns 1997)** requires, when a person is admitted to a penal institution or correctional facility, that proper tests and treatment for a venereal disease are provided.

LA   **La. Rev. Stat. Ann § 15:535 (West 1992 and Supplemental)** authorizes the court to order an adjudicated delinquent or a person convicted of a sexual offense to submit to an STD or HIV test. Requires the procedure or test to be performed by a qualified physician who is required to report any positive result to the Department of Public Safety and Corrections. Requires notification of the test results to the victim or the parent, regardless of the results.

LA   **La. Criminal Procedure Ann. art. 499 (West Supplemental)** requires a person charged by a grand jury for a sexual offense to undergo a medical procedure or tests for STDs and HIV/AIDS. Allows the court to provide the results of the test to the victim and the health authorities. Prohibits the state from using the fact that the test was performed on the alleged offender and the test results in any criminal proceedings arising from the alleged offense.

MT   **Mont. Code Ann. § 50-18-108 (1997)** allows any person confined or imprisoned in any state, county or municipal prison to be examined for an STD. Requires the infected person be treated by health authorities.

NJ   **N.J. Stat. Ann. § 26:4-49.7 (West 1996)** requires the court to order a person who is suspected of being infected with a venereal disease and who is coming before the court on any charge to submit to an examination and treatment.

NJ   **N.J. Stat. Ann. § 26:4-49.8 (West 1996)** requires examining and treating a prisoner for a venereal disease. Allows a prisoner be isolated when a prisoner refuses treatment for a venereal disease. Requires the warden to notify the department when a prisoner with a venereal disease will be released. Requires the notification to be five days prior to the actual date of release or no later than the day following the release date.

ND   **N.D. Cent. Code § 23-07-08 (1991)** requires every person convicted of a crime who is imprisoned for 15 days or more in a state, county or city prison to be examined and treated for STDs.

ND   **N.D. Cent. Code § 23-07-09 (1991)** requires prison authorities of any state, county or city prison to make available a portion of the prison for isolating and treating a person infected with an STD.

OK   **Okla. Stat. Ann. tit. 63, § 1-523 (1997)** requires all correctional facilities, public or private, to have records showing all STD- and HIV-infected inmates and to keep these records on hand for one year. Requires all institutions to furnish a physician with medicine to properly treat an infected person. Requires that facilities provide all correctional employees, probation and parole officers who will have direct contact with inmates, with names of any HIV-infected inmates.

OK   **Okla. Stat. Ann. tit. 63, § 1-524 (1997)** requires examining all prisoners to determine if a prisoner is infected with an STD. Allows a licensed physician to examine persons who are arrested for prostitution or other sex crimes. Allows a person to be detained until the results are known. Requires any person found to be infected with an STD to be treated. Requires quarantining any person who refuses treatment. Requires a person who is arrested for rape and other serious sexual crimes be tested for STDs and HIV. Authorizes the court to issue an order for testing during the arraignment. Requires the order not to include the name and address of the alleged victim. Requires the alleged victim be notified of the test results.

SC   **S.C. Code Ann. § 44-29-100 (Law. Co-op 1997)** authorizes health authorities to examine or treat any person who is imprisoned in any state, county or city prison. Requires a person who, after serving his or her sentence, is suffering from an STD, be isolated and treated at public expense. Allows for a person to report for treatment to a licensed physician at public expense.

SD   **S.D. Codified Laws Ann. § 34-23-6 (1994)** requires all persons imprisoned or confined in any state, county or city prison to be examined and treated for venereal diseases.

SD   **S.D. Codified Laws Ann. § 34-23-7 (1994)** allows health authorities to use any state, county or city prison for isolating and treating a prisoner with a venereal disease.

UT   **Utah Code Ann. § 26-6-19 (1995)** requires an STD-infected person confined in any state, county or city prison to be examined and treated. Requires prison authorities to make a room available for the person suffering with the venereal disease and for them to be isolated and treated at the public's expense. Allows the department to require the person suffering from a venereal disease after imprisonment to report for treatment at the public's expense.

VT   **Vt. Stat. Ann. tit. 13, § 2634 (1974)** requires medical treatment to a person convicted of prostitution and infected with a venereal disease be given before probation or parole to prevent the spread of such disease.

VA   **Va. Code § 32.1-58 (1997)** requires a person convicted of prostitution, soliciting a prostitute or certain sexual crimes be examined and tested for a venereal disease and treated if infected.

VA   **Va. Code § 32.1-59 (1997)** requires any person admitted to any state correctional institution or state hospital to be examined and tested for a venereal disease. Requires the institution to provide treatment and report the case.

WV   **W. Va. Code § 16-4-5 (1995)** requires testing and treating any person who has been convicted of a sexual offense or sexual immorality. Requires not releasing any convicted person from custody until a local health officer has been notified and proper venereal disease tests have been given.

WY   **Wyo. Stat. § 35-4-132 (1997)** requires a physician, other health care provider, administrator of a hospital, dispensary, charitable or penal institution, who diagnoses or treats an STD case, to report the diagnosis to the department and the appropriate health officer. Requires all labs with positive laboratory STD tests to report the diseases. Requires health care providers and facilities to cooperate with and assist the department and health officers in preventing the spread of STDs. Requires the department to compile the number of reported cases within the state.

WY   **Wyo. Stat. § 35-4-134 (1997)** authorizes a health officer to examine, treat and isolate a prisoner confined at any state, county or city jail. Requires providing minimum care and treatment of the individual infected with a incurable STD. Requires examination and treatment of prisoners.

Testing—Premarital Syphilis Testing

(Note: See also Testing—Pregnant Women and Newborns and Testing—Syphilis.)

AL   **Ala. Code § 22-11A-15 (1997)** requires a syphilis examination for a marriage license. Authorizes the Board of Health to charge a reasonable fee for testing. Makes it a Class C misdemeanor for physicians, ministers and others who fail to comply with procedures. Waives requirements for an emergency situation and defines an emergency.

AK   **Alaska Stat. § 18.15.160** requires serological testing for syphilis be performed at approved laboratories of the department and free of charge.

CA   **Cal. Family Code App. § 4300 (West 1994)** requires premarital testing for syphilis not more than 30 days prior to the issuance of a marriage license. Requires a certificate of examination be submitted that states whether the person is infected or not infected with syphilis, or is not infectious to the marital partner.

CT   **Conn. Gen. Stat. § 46b-26 (1997)** requires a test for syphilis and rubella be given before any marriage license is granted.

DC   **D. C. Stat. Code Ann. § 30-117 (1997)** requires a premarital blood test for syphilis before any marriage license can be granted. Requires a doctor's statement declaring that the person applying for the license is not infected with syphilis or is in a stage of the disease that cannot be transmitted to another person.

DC   **D. C. Stat. Code Ann. § 30-118 (1997)** allows a judge to waive the syphilis test for a marriage license.

DC   **D. C. Stat. Code Ann. § 30-119 (1997)** allows a medical officer with the department to conduct a syphilis test and provide a statement needed for a marriage license at no cost when the person is unable to pay due to financial reasons.

DC   **D. C. Stat. Code Ann. § 30-120 (1997)** requires information about a syphilis laboratory blood test required for a marriage license be confidential by any person, agency or committee who obtains, transmits or receives any information.

DC   **D. C. Stat. Code Ann. § 30-121 (1997)** makes it unlawful for any person who knowingly divulges any information about a premarital syphilis blood test, misrepresents or falsifies any facts about a premarital syphilis blood test, issues a marriage license without having received the syphilis-free statement by a licensed physician or fails to comply with taking a required syphilis test for a marriage license. Makes it punishable with a fine of $250, or imprisonment for no more than 6 months, or both.

GA   **Ga. Code Ann. § 19-3-40 (1991)** requires a blood test for syphilis 30 days prior to issuing a marriage license. Allows for free testing if the applicant is unable to pay. Requires a physician's certificate stating whether the applicant is infected or not infected. Outlines the procedure for granting a marriage license when the test is positive and partners are aware of the test results. Any judge, applicant or physician who violates the law by making a false statement is guilty of a misdemeanor.

NJ   **N.J. Stat. Ann. § 37:1-20 (West 1968)** requires an authorized person to have on file, before issuing a marriage license, a certificate signed by a physician that states that the applicant submitted to an approved serological test for syphilis and whether the applicant is or is not infected, or is not in a state when the disease is likely to be communicable. Allows for a statement from the physician in lieu of a certificate.

OK   **Okla. Stat. Ann. tit. 43, § 31 (1990)** requires a premarital examination for syphilis. Requires any person seeking a marriage license to first file with the court clerk a certificate from a physician stating a standard serological exam for syphilis was given. Requires the certificate be used within 30 days of applying for a license.

OK   **Okla. Stat. Ann. tit. 43, § 32 (1990)** outlines the procedure for a judge ordering an extension of no more than 90 days for using a doctor's certificate stating that a premarital exam for syphilis was completed for a marriage license. Requires the judge to be satisfied that both parties are of no harm to society.

OK   **Okla. Stat. Ann. tit. 43, § 37 (1990)** makes it a misdemeanor for any marriage license applicant, physician, governmental employee or laboratory representative to misrepresent any facts or break confidentiality about any syphilis record or lab report.

PA   **Pa. Cons. Stat. Ann. tit. 23, § 1305 (Purdon 1991)** requires a premarital test for syphilis. Requires no marriage license be issued until a statement signed by a licensed physician has been filed. Requires the statement include whether a syphilis test was given and the result from the laboratory. Requires using the physician's statement within 30 days of issuance for the marriage license. Requires a standard serological test for syphilis be a test approved by the department and be made at an approved laboratory. Requires the test be made free of charge when the applicant is unable to pay and when requested by a physician. Allows for an applicant to appeal to the department when having been denied a physician's statement. Outlines filing requirements for marriage licenses and requires all documents be confidential.

PA   **Pa. Cons. Stat. Ann. tit. 35, § 521.12 (Purdon 1993)** makes it unlawful for a physician or representative from a laboratory to misrepresent any facts regarding a premarital examination for syphilis.

WV   **W. Va. Code § 48-1-6 (1996)** requires a marriage application to include the information that a standard serological test for syphilis has been conducted no more than 30 days prior to the date of issuing any marriage license. Requires a statement from the physician stating that the applicant is either not infected with syphilis or is not in a communicable state of infection.

Testing—Syphilis Testing

(Note: See Testing--Pregnant Women and Newborns Section for additional syphilis testing statutes.)

CA   **Cal. Family Code § 4300 (West 19xx)** requires premarital testing for syphilis not more than 30 days prior to the issuance of a marriage license. Requires a certificate of examination to be submitted that states whether the person is infected or not infected with syphilis, or is not infectious to the marital partner.

HI   **Hawaii Rev. Stat. § 325-53 (1993)** requires a report accompany the birth or death certificate that states a woman who gave birth to a child was tested for syphilis. States that failure to test or report for syphilis may be punishable up to a $1,000 fine per violation.

ID   **Idaho Code § 39-1003 (1993)** defines a "standard serological test for syphilis" as a standard serological test for syphilis by the department.

ID   **Idaho Code § 39-1005 (1993)** requires a report on the birth certificate to state whether the woman who bore the child has been tested for syphilis. Prohibits stating the test result on birth or death certificate.

IN   **Ind. Code Ann. § 16-41-14-5 (Burns 1993)** requires the practitioner to test each semen donor for syphilis, Hepatitis B and HIV before the donor provides a donation. Requires a practitioner to test each recipient initially and at least annually as long as artificial insemination procedures are continuing. Requires a practitioner to report all positive results to the department.

IN   **Ind. Code Ann. § 16-41-14-11 (Burns 1993)** specifies that a practitioner or other authorized person is not required to perform any tests for HIV, syphilis or Hepatitis B on a donor's semen if the semen has been previously tested as required, and evidence is submitted that the donor has been tested and all tests were negative.

MA   **Mass. Gen. Laws, Ann. ch. 111, § 121A (West 1996)** requires a physician attending a pregnant woman to take a blood sample during the first examination and submit the sample for a standard serological test for syphilis to a laboratory approved by the department.

ME   **Me. Rev. Stat. Ann. tit. 22, § 1232 (1992)** authorizes the department to approve one or more tests for syphilis. Allows the department to approve and appoint other laboratories in addition to the state laboratory to make a syphilis test. Requires that with every positive syphilis test, the name, address, age and sex of the person be reported to the department.

MT   **Mont. Code Ann. § 50-18-104 (1997)** requires the department to approve a standard serological test for syphilis and to approve laboratories that may make the test. Requires the department to allow for a test when requested.

MT   **Mont. Code Ann. § 50-19-104 (1997)** requires the test for syphilis be done at the department laboratory or a laboratory approved by the department.

MT   **Mont. Code Ann. § 50-19-109 (1997)** allows a person to waive the requirement for a syphilis test due to religious beliefs.

NJ   **N.J. Stat. Ann. § 26:4-49.2 (West 1996)** requires standard serological tests for syphilis be performed in a state laboratory without charge.

NJ   **N.J. Stat. Ann. § 26:4-49.6 (West 1996)** requires a migrant laborer to submit to a syphilis, gonorrhea and venereal disease examination within 30 days after entering New Jersey to work, unless the migrant laborer can prove that a venereal disease was completed within the last 90 days. Requires any person who employs a migrant laborer to notify the state department of health within five days of the beginning of employment whether the person has been examined for a venereal disease.

NC   **N.C. Gen. Stat. § 15A-615 (1997)** allows testing a sex offender who has had an alleged sexual contact with any minor under age 16 for STDs including chlamydia, gonorrhea, Hepatitis B. herpes, HIV and syphilis. Allows the victim to petition the court for the offender to be tested. Requires the test results be reported to the local health director. Requires the victim and alleged offender be informed of the test results and provided with counseling. Requires the results of the test not be admissible as evidence in any criminal proceeding.

OK   **Okla. Stat. Ann. tit. 43, § 34 (1990)** requires the state provide syphilis examinations free of charge if requested by the patient.

OK   **Okla. Stat. Ann. tit. 43, § 35 (1990)** requires all standard serological tests for syphilis be conducted at a laboratory approved by the state and be completed free of charge if requested by the person tested.

VT   **Vt. Stat. Ann. tit. 18, § 1104 (1982)** defines a "serological syphilis test" as a test approved by the board and performed by the state laboratory.

WA   **Wash. Rev. Code Ann. § 70.24.100 (1996)** standardizes syphilis laboratory tests. Requires a standard serological test be a laboratory test for syphilis approved by the secretary of health and be performed either by a laboratory approved by the secretary or by the department. Requires tests be free of charge at the request of the physician.

Treatment—Other

AL   **Ala. Code § 22-11A-13 (1997)** authorizes and directs the Board of Health to declare rules for testing, reporting, investigation and treatment of STDs.

AL   **Ala. Code § 22-11A-23 (1997)** requires any person be tested who the state or county health officer has reason to believe has been exposed to STDs. Requires any person who the state or county health officer has reason to believe is infected with STDs to seek and accept treatment at the direction of the health officer or a licensed physician.

AL   **Ala. Code § 22-11A-24 (1997)** allows a state or county health officer to petition a probate judge of the county to commit a person to the custody of the department for compulsory testing, for treatment or quarantine, when any person who is exposed to an STD or where reasonable evidence indicates exposure to an STD, refuses testing or treatment, or whose conduct indicates exposure to others.

CA   **Cal. Health & Safety Code § 120565 (West 1996)** allows an agency to investigate whether a person who has discontinued treatment has initiated or is participating in treatment elsewhere.

CA   **Cal. Health & Safety Code § 120570 (West 1996)** requires an agency to report to the department the name of a person who refuses to comply with treatment.

CO   **Colo. Rev. Stat. § 25-4-406 (1997)** requires the department to make rules and regulations providing for the quarantine, treatment and control of venereal diseases. Requires all department rules and regulations regarding venereal diseases to have the effect of law.

CO   **Colo. Rev. Stat. § 25-4-408 (1997)** requires the department to prepare and distribute free information about the dangers of venereal diseases, how to prevent them, and the necessity for treatment. Requires any physician who examines or treats a person with a venereal disease to instruct the infected person on how to prevent the spread of the disease, the necessity for treatment and to give a free copy of information regarding venereal diseases.

DE   **Del. Code Ann. tit. 16, § 703 (1996)** authorizes the director to isolate, examine, investigate and treat any person suspected of being infected with STDs. Authorizes the director to require a person infected with an STD to find treatment.

DE   **Del. Code Ann. tit. 16, § 704 (1996)** establishes the procedure for the apprehension, commitment, treatment, quarantine and possible court hearings of an STD-infected person. Sets guidelines for anyone who refuses to comply. Allows the director of the Division of Public Health to petition the courts for an order to quarantine and treat an infected person. Outlines the procedures.

DE   **Del. Code Ann. tit. 16, § 705 (1996)** outlines emergency public health procedures for suspected or infected persons who refuse testing, examination or treatment and who present a threat to the public health. Allows the director of the Division of Public Health to ask the court for an injunction or to take the infected person into custody.

DE   **Del. Code Ann. tit. 16, § 707 (1996)** authorizes the department to make rules and regulations in regard to reporting, controlling and treating people with STDs.

FL   **Fla. Stat. Ann. § 384.28 (West 1993 and Supplemental 1998)** requires specific protocol be followed when attempting hospitalization, placement and treatment for an STD-infected person who is considered a threat to the public health. Allows the department to petition a court order for the hospitalization and treatment of an infected person. Prohibits placing a person under age 18 in a hospital or in another health care facility where adults are hospitalized.

FL   **Fla. Stat. Ann. § 384.284 (West 1993)** requires the department to develop and supply all necessary forms to be used by the circuit court for ordering the physical examination, treatment and hospitalization of an STD-infected person.

FL   **Fla. Stat. Ann. § 384.288 (West 1993 and Supplemental 1998)** outlines fees and other compensation for services required during the hospitalization, physical examination and treatment of a person infected with an STD.

FL   **Fla. Stat. Ann. § 384.33 (West 1993)** allows the department to adopt rules regarding the investigation, treatment and confidentiality of STDs.

ID   **Idaho Code § 39-601A (1993)** requires governmental authorities to provide services authorized or mandated by the law for treating or testing venereal diseases only to the extent of funding and available resources appropriate.

ID   **Idaho Code § 39-605 (1993)** authorizes the state Board of Health and Welfare to make rules concerning the control, treatment and quarantine of persons infected with a venereal disease.

IL   **Ill. Ann. Stat. ch. 410 § 325/10 (Smith-Hurd 1997)** requires the department to adopt the rules necessary to performing the duties of the department. Requires rules of the department to include criteria, standards and procedures for the identification, investigation, examination and treatment of STDs.

IN   **Ind. Code Ann. § 16-41-15-17 (Burns 1993)** allows for a religious exemption for treating a venereal disease.

IA   **Iowa Code § 140.14 (1997)** allows for a religious exemption for the testing and treatment of a venereal disease.

LA   **La. Rev. Stat. Ann § 1066 (West 1992)** makes it unlawful for a person to sell any drug for the treatment of a venereal disease unless prescribed by a licensed physician.

LA   **La. Rev. Stat. Ann § 1067 (West 1992)** requires the secretary of the department to make rules and regulations for the diagnosis, treatment, reporting and prevention of venereal diseases.

MA   **Mass. Gen. Laws Ann. ch. 111, § 117 (West 1996)** requires the department, along with cooperation from local boards or hospitals, establish and maintain clinics for treating venereal diseases for any person unable to pay. Allows cities and towns to establish clinics through their boards. Requires treatment in a clinic to include providing transportation or the reasonable cost of transportation to and from the place for the patient who is unable to pay.

MA   **Mass. Gen. Laws Ann. ch. 111, § 118 (West 1996)** requires that no discrimination be made against a person who is receiving treatment for a venereal disease in a hospital supported by city taxes.

MI   **Mich. Stat. Ann. § 14.15 (5111) (Law. Co-op 1995)** authorizes the department to establish reporting requirements for serious communicable diseases. Allows the department to require a licensed health professional or health facility to report a serious communicable disease or infection within 24 hours of diagnosis. Requires local health departments to furnish care for tuberculosis and venereal diseases. Requires the department to provide rules for the confidentiality of reports, records and data pertaining to the testing, care, treatment, reporting and research associated with tuberculosis, Hepatitis B and other venereal diseases.

MI   **Mich. Stat. Ann. § 14.15 (5117) (Law. Co-op 1995)** requires the local health department to provide medical care for any person with a serious communicable disease or infection, including tuberculosis and any venereal disease. Requires the local department to report the case to the individual's county department of social services.

MN   **Minn. Stat. § 144.065 (1996)** requires the state commissioner of health to assist local health agencies and organizations to develop services for the detection and treatment of venereal diseases. Requires these agencies to provide services for the diagnosis and treatment of venereal diseases and provide appropriate educational information. Requires the state commissioner to provide rules and technical assistance on providing services and establish a method of providing funds to these agencies.

MN   **Minn. Stat. § 62Q.14 (1996)** prohibits any health insurance plan from restricting the choice of an enrollee as to where the enrollee receives services related to testing and treatment of STDs.

MS   **Miss. Code Ann. § 1-23-30 (1993)** requires the county health departments to provide free testing and treatment for STDs. Requires all testing and treatment be held confidential. Requires using available media to advertise the confidentiality of the test and treatment.

MO   **Mo. Ann. Stat. § 431.061** allows a minor under age 18 to consent to treatment for a venereal disease.

MT   **Mont. Code Ann. § 50-18-102 (1997)** authorizes the department to prevent, control and prescribe treatment for STDs and to conduct educational campaigns.

MT   **Mont. Code Ann. § 50-18-103 (1997)** requires the department to cooperate with federal agencies regarding the prevention, control and treatment of STDs. Allows the department to expend federal funds made available to the state for the prevention, control and treatment of STDs.

MT   **Mont. Code Ann. § 50-18-110 (1997)** makes it unlawful to prescribe, sell or recommend any drugs, medicines or other substances for the cure or alleviation of an STD except by a prescription signed by a legally authorized person.

NV   **Nev. Rev. Stat. § 441A.240 (1993)** requires the health division to control, prevent, treat and, whenever possible, ensure the cure of STDs. Requires the health division to provide materials and the curriculum necessary to conduct an educational program and to establish a program for the certification of persons qualified to instruct the program.

NV   **Nev. Rev. Stat. § 441A.250 (1993)** allows the health division to establish and provide financial assistance or other support to clinics and dispensaries for the prevention, control, and treatment or cure of STDs.

NV   **Nev. Rev. Stat. § 441A.260 (1993)** allows the health divisions to provide medical supplies and financial aid for the STD treatment of indigent patients. Requires physicians, clinics or dispensaries that accept supplies or aid to comply with all conditions prescribed by the board.

NV   **Nev. Rev. Stat. § 441A.280 (1993)** requires a physician or clinic to attempt to persuade an infected person to submit to medical treatment. Authorizes a physician or clinic to notify the health authority if that person does not submit to treatment, or does not complete the prescribed course of treatment.

NJ   **N.J. Stat. Ann. § 26:4-29 (West 1996)** requires a venereal disease case to be regarded as infectious until a licensed physician has examined the person and stated otherwise.

NJ   **N.J. Stat. Ann. § 26:4-46 (West 1996)** allows any person who is suffering from a venereal disease and who is unable to pay for treatment to apply for care and treatment. Requires the board to pay for treatment when a person is unable to pay.

NJ   **N.J. Stat. Ann. § 26:4-47 (West 1996)** allows free diagnosis and treatment of STDs to be provided by the state Department of Health. Allows the commissioner of health to establish rules and regulations pertaining to the payment for services and educational materials provided by the department.

NM   **N. M. Stat. Ann. § 24-1-9 (1997)** allows any person, regardless of age, to consent to an examination and treatment by a licensed physician for an STD.

NY   **N.Y. Public Health Law § 2304 (McKinney 1993)** requires that the Board of Health provide adequate facilities for the free diagnosis and treatment of persons suspected of being infected or who are infected with an STD. Authorizes the health officer to administer these facilities. Allows a person to be treated at his own expense by a licensed physician of his choice. Requires facilities to comply with the requirements of the commissioner.

NY   **N.Y. Public Health Law § 2305 (McKinney 1993)** prohibits any person other than a licensed physician from diagnosing, treating or prescribing medicine to a person infected with an STD. Allows a licensed physician to diagnose, treat, or prescribe for a person under age 21 without the consent or knowledge of a parent or guardian.

NY   **N.Y. Public Health Law § 2308-a (McKinney 1993)** requires the administrative officer or other person in charge of a health clinic providing medical treatment for women, to offer every resident coming to such clinics or facilities for treatment, appropriate examinations or tests for the detection of STDs.

ND   **N.D. Cent. Code § 23-07-07 (1991)** authorizes the state, local and city health officers, when necessary for the protection of public health, to examine any person suspected of being infected with an STD, to require any person to report for treatment, to investigate any cases and to cooperate with other officials to enforce the laws.

OH   **Ohio Rev. Code Ann. § 3709. 24 (Page 1997)** allows a board of health of any city or general health district to set up clinics to provide free treatment for gonorrhea, syphilis and chancroid. Allows these clinics to be used for quarantining cases of gonorrhea, syphilis and chancroid or other cases the director of health orders to be quarantined.

OK   **Okla. Stat. Ann. tit. 63, § 1-519 (1997)** makes it a felony for an infected person, before being discharged and pronounced cured in writing by a physician, to marry or to expose any person to a venereal disease.

OK   **Okla. Stat. Ann. tit. 63, § 1-520 (1997)** makes it a misdemeanor for any physician who discharges an STD-infected person early from treatment or provides a written statement stating an infected person is noninfectious.

OK   **Okla. Stat. Ann. tit. 63, § 1-521 (1997)** makes it unlawful for any person who is not a physician to treat an STD-infected person for pay unless acting under the direction of a physician.

OK   **Okla. Stat. Ann. tit. 63, § 1-522 (1997)** makes it unlawful for any person to offer or provide treatment, sell or furnish any medication to an STD infected person without a prescription.

PA   **Pa. Cons. Stat. Ann. tit. 35, § 521.8 (Purdon 1993)** allows any person taken into custody and charged with a sex offense crime to be examined for a venereal disease by a department or court-appointed physician. Allows any person convicted of a crime and suspected of being infected to be examined for a venereal disease. Requires treating any person found to be infected with a venereal disease.

PA   **Pa. Cons. Stat. Ann. tit. 35, 521.9 (Purdon 1993)** requires the department to provide free diagnosis and treatment for anyone with a venereal disease. Allows any local board or department to share in the financial support for providing free diagnosis and treatment for a venereal disease.

PA   **Pa. Cons. Stat. Ann. tit. 35, § 521.10 (Purdon 1993)** requires drugs be sold for treatment of a venereal disease only with a prescription from a licensed physician.

RI   **R.I. Gen. Laws § 23-11-4 (1996)** authorizes the department to establish a reasonable fee structure for state laboratory tests and clinical treatments.

RI   **R.I. Gen. Laws § 23-11-10 (1996)** authorizes the department to take appropriate measures to investigate sources of STD infections. Allows full powers for the inspection, examination and treatment of all suspected STD cases and sources.

SD   **S.D. Codified Laws Ann. § 34-23-13 (1994)** requires the state department to make rules and regulations concerning the care, treatment and quarantine of persons infected with a venereal disease.

TN   **Tenn. Code Ann. § 68-10-103 (1996)** requires a physician or other person treating persons infected with an STD to provide information regarding STDs. Requires the information be furnished by the department.

VT   **Vt. Stat. Ann. tit. 18, § 1096 (1982)** makes it a violation for any person infected with a venereal disease to refuse treatment, with a fine of no more than $500, or imprisonment for no more than six months, or both.

VT   **Vt. Stat. Ann. tit. 18, § 1098 (1982)** requires the board to provide free testing for suspected venereal disease cases and provide free hospitalization and other treatment for infected patients who are unable to pay. Requires the board not to pay for the diagnosis and treatment until all required reports are completed by the physician and supplied to the board.

VT   **Vt. Stat. Ann. tit. 18, § 1100 (1982)** requires the board to make and enforce any rule or regulation for quarantining and treating any reported venereal disease cases for the protection of the public.

VA   **Va. Code § 32.1-56 (1997)** requires a physician or any other person who examines or treats a person having a venereal disease to provide information to the infected person about the disease, the nature of the disease, methods of treatment, prevention of the spread of the disease, and the necessity of tests to ensure that a cure has been accomplished.

VA   **Va. Code § 32.1-59 (1997)** requires any person admitted to any state correctional institution or state hospital be examined and tested for a venereal disease. Requires the institution to provide treatment and report the case.

WA   **Wash. Rev. Code Ann. § 70.24.095 (1996)** requires a health care practitioner attending a pregnant woman or attending a drug treatment program participant who is seeking treatment of an STD to ensure that the patient receives AIDS counseling.

WV   **W. Va. Code § 16-4-9 (1995)** requires a physician or other person who examines or treats a person with syphilis, gonorrhea or chancroid, to inform that person of the necessity of taking treatment and continuing the treatment as prescribed. Requires a physician to report a patient who has stopped treatment to the local health officer. Makes it a misdemeanor for anyone to stop treatment for a venereal disease. Requires the local health officer to investigate any unfinished treatments for a venereal disease. Authorizes the local health officer to arrest, detain, and quarantine any patient who fails to return for treatment.

WV   **W. Va. Code § 16-4-19 (1995)** allows a person to voluntary submit to an examination and treatment for a venereal disease. Allows the person to receive treatment at a local clinic free of charge if that person is unable to pay.

WV   **W. Va. Code § 16-4-24 (1995)** makes it a misdemeanor for a druggist or other person who is not a licensed physician to prescribe, recommend or sell any medicine to be used for treating syphilis, gonorrhea or chancroid.

WI   **Wis. Stat. Ann. § 252.10 (West Supplemental 1997)** requires programs in counties with an incidence of gonorrhea, chlamydia, or syphilis that exceed the statewide average, to diagnose and treat STDs at no cost to the patient. Requires the county board of supervisors to be responsible for ensuring that the program exists, but are required to establish their own programs only if no other public or private program is operating. Requires the department to compile statistics indicating the incidence of gonorrhea, chlamydia and syphilis for each county in the state.

WY   **Wyo. Stat. § 35-4-130 (1997)** makes it a misdemeanor for any person violating or refusing to comply with the rules and regulations regarding STD testing, treatment and reporting, and is punishable by a fine of no more than $750, imprisonment for no more than six months, or both.

Appendix A

Division of STD Prevention Activities

The following Centers for Disease Control and Prevention STD prevention and control activities are conducted through the Division of Sexually Transmitted Disease Prevention.[55]

STD Morbidity and Behavioral Surveillance

The CDC collects and organizes national data on STD rates. It also collects STD-related behavioral data from state and local STD control programs, prevalence monitoring systems, health care utilization surveys, and reproductive health and behavior surveys. STD surveillance is extremely challenging for the CDC because STDs account for at least 79 percent of all nationally notifiable diseases reported to the CDC in 1995 alone.

Infertility Prevention Program

The collaborative efforts occurring in infertility prevention represent only the fourth nationwide STD prevention program in U.S. history, including the nationwide HIV prevention program. The infertility prevention program focuses on 1) the Regional Infertility Prevention Projects 2) applied infertility research and, 3) the development of chlamydia screening guidelines for the managed care Health Plan Employer Data Information Set (HEDIS).

Syphilis Prevention Research Program

Syphilis remains a major public health problem in the United States, especially among minority populations. The southern states have the highest rates of syphilis. The program, Innovations in Syphilis Prevention in the United States: Reconsidering the Epidemiology and Involving Communities, was initiated in 1995. The mission of the program is to develop innovative, practical and community-involved STD prevention programs; to foster intramural and extramural collaboration on major prevention research; to implement research and development projects for syphilis elimination in the United States; and to build collaborative intervention partnerships with communities that are affected by syphilis.

Research on STD/HIV Interactions

Research on the interactions of STDs and HIV infection are useful to determine the effect of STDs on HIV transmission and acquisition, as well as to understand the effect of HIV infection on other STD clinical presentations, diagnosis and treatment. Studies show there is strong scientific evidence that supports the idea that other STDs facilitate sexual transmission of HIV infection, and that HIV infection affects the clinical course of other STDs. The evidence makes a strong case for enhancing STD control activities as a critical component of HIV prevention activities.

Accelerated Prevention Campaign Projects

One component of the STD Accelerated Prevention Campaign (APC) is called the Enhanced Projects. This project enables state health departments to implement and evaluate new, locally relevant approaches to STD prevention beyond the traditional, clinic-based model. Local resources have to provide a $1 match for every $2 provided by the federal government. The goals of the program include providing innovative STD prevention programs and developing more cost-effective means of STD prevention.

Intervention Research to Reduce Risky Behaviors

This project focuses on long-term behavior change as a method of preventing STDs. The research focuses on finding why people make the decisions they do in situations that can effect their health, such as sexual behavior.

Research on Seeking and Providing Health Care

CDC funds four projects that are designed to answer questions surrounding screening, treatment, prevention and provider efforts in the field of STDs.

International Activities

CDC participates in international research endeavors if the outcome is applicable to the United States and the host country sees that the CDC has an important role to play. Countries currently or previously involved in research efforts include Bolivia, the Central African Republic, the Caribbean, Cote d'Ivoire, Indonesia, Jamaica, the Republic of South Africa, and Uganda.

STD Prevention in Correctional Facilities

The CDC is addressing the need to focus on hard-to-reach, high-risk populations in correctional facilities by trying to increase the early detection and treatment of women in correctional facilities who are infected with syphilis, gonorrhea and chlamydia. A rapid syphilis screening and treatment program has been implemented in Chicago's Cook County Jail. Other implementations are taking place in Greenville, Mississippi; New York City; Los Angeles County; and Nassau County, New York.

STD Hotline

The National STD Hotline is toll-free and available nationwide. Trained information specialists provide callers with current STD prevention information and referrals.

Provider Training

One of the more critical components of STD prevention and control is to ensure that clinicians are skilled in STD diagnosis and treatment. CDC supports the training of providers of STD services through training centers, programs and fellowships.

Appendix B

State STD Program Managers

Mike O'Cain
Division of STD Control
Department of Public Health
RSA Tower, Suite 1450
P.O. Box 303017
Montgomery, AL 36130-3017
(334) 206-5350
(334) 206-2090 (fax)

Wendy Craytor
Department of Health and Social Services
3601 C Street, Suite 540
P.O. Box 240249
Anchorage, AK 99524-0249
(907) 269-8058
(907) 561-4239 (fax)

Tai Ripley, R.N.
STD Control Program
Department of Health
LBJ Tropical Medical Center
P.O. Box F
Pago Pago, AS 96799
9-011-(684) 633-4606
9-011-(684) 633-5379 (fax)

Frank Slaughter
Office of HIV/STD Services
Arizona Department of Health Services
3815 North Black Canyon Highway
Phoenix, AZ 85015
(602) 230-5905
(602) 230-5818 (fax)

Arlene Rose
Director, Division of AIDS/STD
Department of Health
4815 West Markham, Room 453, Slot 33
Little Rock, AR 72205-3867
(501) 661-2665
(501) 661-2082 (fax)

Tom Ault
Department of Health Services
601 North 7th Street, MS 460
P.O. Box 942732
Sacramento, CA 94234-7320
(916) 323-1457
(916) 322-5447 (fax)

A. Michael Lawrence, M.P.A.
Preventive Health Services
County of Los Angeles
2615 South Grand Avenue, Room 500
Los Angeles, CA 90007
(213) 744-3085
(213) 749-9606 (fax)

Wendy Wolf, M.P.A.
City Clinic
San Francisco Department of Public Health
356 7th Street
San Francisco, CA 94103
(415) 487-5501
(415) 495-6463 (fax)

Nancy Spencer, M.P.H.
STD/AIDS Field Services Section
DCEED-STD-A3
Colorado Department of Health and Environment
4300 Cherry Creek Drive, South
Denver, CO 80222
(303) 692-2741
(303) 782-5393 (fax)

Ted Pestorius
STD Program
Department of Public Health
410 Capitol Avenue, MS 11STD
P.O. Box 340308
Hartford, CT 06134-0308
(860) 509-7920
(860) 509-7743 (fax)

John Health
STD Control Program
Department of Health
717 14th Street, N.W., Suite 950
Washington, DC 20005
(202) 727-9853
(202) 727-3345 (fax)

Jack E. Wroten
Chief
Florida Bureau of STD Control and Prevention
1317 Winewood Boulevard
Building 6, Room 414E
Tallahassee, FL 32399-0700
850) 921-1521
(850) 487-3687 (fax)

Mark Schrader
Director, STD/HIV Program
Georgia Department of Human Resources
2 Peachtree Street
10th Floor, Suite 400
Atlanta, GA 30303-3186
(404) 657-3100
(404) 657-3133 (fax)

Josie O'Mallan
STD/HIV Coordinator
Bureau of Communicable Disease Control
Government of Guam
P.O. Box 2816
Agana, GU 96910
9-011 (671) 735-2852
9-011 (671) 734-5910 (fax)

Roy Ohye
STD/HIV Prevention Program
Department of Health
3627 Kilauea Avenue, Room 304
Honolulu, HI 96816-2399
(808) 733-9287
(808) 733-9291 (fax)

Anne Williamson, M.H.E.
STD/AIDS Program Manager
Bureau of Clinical and Preventive Services
Department of Health and Welfare
450 West State Street, 4th Floor
Boise, ID 83720
(208) 334-6526
(208) 332-7346 (fax)

Charles Rabins, M.P.H.
Acting Chief, Division of Infectious Disease
Illinois Department of Public Health
525 West Jefferson Street
Springfield, IL 62761
(217) 782-2747
(217) 524-5443 (fax)

Anne Meegan
13th Street Specialty Clinic
Department of Health
1306 South Michigan Avenue, 2nd Floor
Chicago, IL 60605
(312) 747-0120
(312) 747-0160 (fax)

Jim Beall
Division of HIV/STD
Indiana State Department of Health
2 North Meridian Street
P.O. Box 1964
Indianapolis, IN 46204
(317) 233-7426
(317) 233-7663 (fax)

John Katz
Division of Health Protection
Department of Public Health
Lucas State Office Building
Des Moines, IA 50319-0075
(515) 281-4936
(515) 281-4570 (fax)

Ron Turski
STD Control Program
Department of Health and Environment
109 S.W. 9th Street
Mills Building, Suite 605
Topeka, KS 66612-1271
(913) 291-3378
(913) 296-4197 (fax)

David Raines
Department of Health Services
Cabinet for Human Resources
275 East Main Street
Frankfort, KY 40621
(502) 564-4804
(502) 564-4553 (fax)

Jim Scioneaux
STD Control Program
Office of Public Health
Department of Health and Hospitals
325 Loyola Avenue, Room 616
New Orleans, LA 70112
(504) 568-5275
(504) 568-5279 (fax)

Bob Woods
Program Manager
STD Program, Bureau of Health
Department of Human Services
State House, Station 11
Augusta, ME 04333
(207) 287-5199
(207) 287-6865 (fax)

Elsie Ramon
Director of Communicable Diseases
Mariana Islands Department of Public Health
  and Environmental Services
P.O. Box 409 CK
Saipan, MP 96950
(670) 234-8950
(670) 234-8930 (fax)

Peter Bien
Ministry of Health Services
Republic of Marshall Islands
P.O. Box 16
Majuro, MH 96960
9-011-(692) 625-3355
9-011-(692) 625-3432 (fax)

Dave Akers
Division of STD Control
Department of Health and Mental Hygiene
3rd Floor, Room 307-B
201 West Preston Street
Baltimore, MD 21201
(410) 225-6684
(410) 333-5529 (fax)

Wayne Brathwalte
Preventive Medicine and Epidemiology
Baltimore City Health Department
210 Guilford Avenue, 3rd Floor
Baltimore, MD 21202
(410) 396-4448
(410) 396-8457 (fax)

Paul Etkind, M.P.H.
STD Control Program
State Laboratory Institute
Department of Public Health
305 South Street
Boston, MA 02130-3597
(617) 983-6941
(617) 983-6962 (fax)

Mark A. Miller
Chief, STD Program
Michigan Department of Community Health
3423 North Martin Luther King Jr. Boulevard
Lansing, MI 48909
(517) 335-8167
(517) 335-8166 (fax)

Kidsen K. Iohp, M.P.H.
Health Program Manager
Department of Health Services
P.O. Box PS 70
Palikir
Pohnpel, FM 96941
9-011-(691) 320-2872
9-011-(691) 320-5263 (fax)

Jill DeBoer, M.P.H.
Manager
AIDS/STD Prevention Services Section
Minnesota Department of Health
717 Delaware Street, S.E.
Box 9441
Minneapolis, MN 55440-9441
(612) 623-5698
(612) 623-5739 (fax)

Mike Cassell
STD Program Manager
STD Control Program
Department of Public Health
P.O. Box 1700
Jackson, MS 39215-1700
(601) 960-7714
(601) 960-7909 (fax)

Mary Hayes
Bureau of STD/HIV Prevention
Department of Health
930 Wildwood
Jefferson City, MO 65109
(573) 751-6141
(573) 751-6417 (fax)

Sally Klein, R.N.
Supervisor, HIV/STD Section
Montana Department of Public Health
Cogswell Building, Room C-305
Helena, MT 59620
(406) 444-9028
(406) 444-2920 (fax)

Dan Harrah
STD Control Program
Division of Disease Control
Department of Health
P.O. Box 95007
Lincoln, NE 68509-5007
(402) 471-2937
(402) 471-6426 (fax)

Robert M. Nellis
Bureau of Disease Control and Intervention Services
Nevada State Health Department
505 East King Street, Room 304
Carson City, NV 89710
(702) 687-4800
(702) 687-4988 (fax)

David R. Ayotte, M.S..P H
STD/HIV Program
Bureau of Disease Control
Division of Public Health Services
6 Hazen Drive
Concord, NH 03301
(603) 271-4502
(603) 271-4934 (fax)

Jerry Carolina
STD Control Program
Division of Epidemiology and Disease Control
State Department of Health
3635 Quakerbridge Road, Box 369
Trenton, NJ 08625-0369
(609) 588-7476
(609) 588-7462 (fax)

Al Chowning, M.P.H.
Public Health Division/STD
Health Department
525 Camino de Los Marquez, Suite 1
Santa Fe, NM 87501
(505) 476-8459
(505) 827-2193 (fax)

Dennis Murphy
STD Control Section
Department of Health
ESP Corning Tower, Room 1168
Albany, NY 12237
(518) 474-3598
(518) 474-3491 (fax)

Steve Rubin
Bureau of STD Control
NYC Department of Health
125 Worth Street
Box 73, Room 207
New York, NY 10013
(212) 788-4413
(212) 788-4431 (fax)

Paul Esbrandt
HIV/STD Prevention and Care Section
Department of Health and Human Services
P.O. Box 29601
Raleigh, NC 27626-0601
(919) 733-9514
(919) 733-1020 (fax)

Kirby Kruger
Division of Disease Control/STD Program
North Dakota Department of Health
State Capitol Building
600 East Boulevard Avenue
Bismarck, ND 58505-0200
(701) 224-2378
(701) 328-1412 (fax)

Juliet C. Dorris-Mason, M.S.W.
Health Planning Administrator
HIV/STD Prevention Program
35 East Chestnut Street, 7th Floor
P.O. Box 118
Columbus, OH 43266-0118
(614) 728-9256
(614) 728-0876 (fax)

Mark Turner
HIV/STD Service, Mail Drop 0308
Oklahoma Department of Health
1000 N.E. 10th Street
Oklahoma City, OK 73117-1299
(405) 271-4636
(405) 271-5149 (fax)

Doug Harger
STD Program
Oregon Health Division
800 N.E. Oregon Street, Suite 745
Portland, OR 97232
(503) 731-4026
(503) 731-4082 (fax)

Caleb T. Otto, M.D.
Chief of Public Health
Ministry of Health
P.O. Box 6027
Koror, PW 96940
(680) 488-3116
(680) 488-3115 (fax)

Martin Goldberg
Division of Disease Control
Department of Public Health
500 South Broad Street
Philadelphia, PA 19146
(215) 875-5637
(215) 545-8362 (fax)

Ed Powers
STD Control
State Department of Health
P.O. Box 90
Harrisburg, PA 17108
(717) 787-3981
(717) 783-3794 (fax)

Nelson Colon-Cartegena
Puerto Rico Department of Health
Pabellom #1 Altos
Old Psychiatric Hospital
Monacillos Medical Center
San Juan, PR 00922
(787) 274-5508
(787) 274-5566 (fax)

Margarita Pagan-Medena
Puerto Rico Department of Health
Pabellon #1 ALTOS
Old Psychiatric Hospital
Monacillos Medical Center
San Juan, PR 00922
(787) 274-5565
(787) 274-5503 (fax)

Janet O'Connell, R.N., M.P.H.
STD Program Manager
Rhode Island Department of Health
Three Capitol Hill, Cannon Building
Providence, RI 02908-5097
(401) 277-1365
(401) 272-3771 (fax)

Tim Lindman
South Carolina Department of Health
  and Environmental Control
Mills/Jarrett Complex
1751 Calhoun Street
Columbia, SC 29201
(803) 737-4110
(803) 737-3979 (fax)

David Morgan
Office of Disease Prevention
Department of Health
615 East 4th Street
Pierre, SD 57501
(605) 773-3737
(605) 773-5509 (fax)

Chris Freeman
STD/HIV Program
Tennessee Department of Health
Cordell Hull Building, 4th Floor
426 Fifth Avenue, North
Nashville, TN 37247
(615) 532-8516
(615) 532-8478 (fax)

Casey S. Blass
HIV/STD Health Resources Division
Bureau of HIV and STD Prevention
1100 West 49th Street
Austin, TX 78756-9987
(512) 490-2515
(512) 490-2538 (fax)

Cristie Chesler
Bureau of Epidemiology
Department of Health
288 North 1460 West
P.O. Box 142870
Salt Lake City, UT 84114-2870
(801) 538-6191
(801) 538-9923 (fax)

Marilyn Richards
STD Control Section
Vermont Department of Health
108 Cherry Street
P.O. Box 70
Burlington, VT 05402
(802) 863-7305
(802) 865-7314 (fax)

Stan Phillips
STD/HIV/TB Program
Virgin Islands Department of Health
48 Sugar Estates
St. Thomas, VI 00801
(809) 774-3168
(809) 777-4001 (fax)

Casey Riley
Bureau of STD/AIDS Control
Department of Health
P.O. Box 2448, Room 112
Richmond, VA 23218
(804) 786-6267
(804) 225-3517 (fax)

Larry Klopfenstein
Director, STD/TB Services
Department of Health
Airdustrial Park, Building 14
P.O. Box 47842
Olympia, WA 98504-7842
(360) 753-5810
(360) 586-5440 (fax)

Robert Johnson
Department of Health and Human Resources
1422 Washington Street, East
Charleston, WV 25301
(304) 558-2950
(304) 558-6335 (fax)

Anthony Wade
Director, STD Program
Division of Health
Department of Health and Family Services
1414 E. Washington Avenue
Madison, WI 53703-3044
(608) 266-7365
(608) 266-2906 (fax)

Roger Burr
STD Prevention Program
Division of Public Health
Branch of Preventive Medicine
Hathaway Building, Room 520
Cheyenne, WY 82002
(307) 777-6013
(307) 777-5279 (fax)

APPENDIX C

STATE STD PROJECT DIRECTORS

Charles H. Woernle, M.D., M.P.H.
Assistant State Health Officer
Alabama Department of Public Health
RSA Tower, Suite 1450
P.O. Box 303017
Montgomery, AL 36130-3017
(334) 206-5325
(334) 206-2090 (fax)

John Middaugh, M.D.
Chief, Section of Epidemiology
Department of Health and Social Services
3601 "C" Street, Suite 540
P.O. Box 240249
Anchorage, AK 99524-0249
(907) 269-8000
(907) 561-6588 (fax)

Joseph Tufa, M.D.
Deputy Director of Health
Department of Health
LBJ Tropical Medical Center
P.O. Box F
Pago Pago, AS 96799
9-011 (684) 633-4590
9-011 (684) 633-1869 (fax)

Chris Brown
Chief, Office of HIV/STD Services
Division of Disease Prevention
3815 North Black Canyon Highway
Phoenix, AZ 85015
(602) 230-5816
(602) 230-5817 (fax)

Martha Hiett
Bureau of Public Health Programs
Arkansas Department of Health
Room 453, Mail Slot #41
4815 West Markham
Little Rock, AR 72205-3867
(501) 661-2243
(501) 661-2055 (fax)

Gary Richwald, M.D., M.P.H.
Medical Director, STD Program
Preventive Health Services
County of Los Angeles
2615 South Grand Avenue, Room 500
Los Angeles, CA 90007-2668
(213) 744-3093
(214) 749-9606 (fax)

Gail Bolan, M.D.
STD Control Branch
2151 Berkeley Way, Room 715
Berkeley, CA 94704
(510) 540-3240
(510) 849-5057 (fax)

Vacant
STD Prevention and Control Section
San Francisco Department of Public Health
1360 Mission Street, Suite 401
San Francisco, CA 94103
(415) 554-8499
(415) 554-9636 (fax)

Ellen Mangione, M.D., M.P.H.
STD/AIDS Section
DCEED-A3
Department of Public Health and Environment
4300 Cherry Creek Drive
Denver, CO 80222
(303) 692-2613
(303) 782-5393 (fax)

James L. Hadler, M.D., M.P.H.
Chief, Epidemiology Section
Department of Public Health
410 Capitol Avenue, MS #11 EPI
P.O. Box 340308
Hartford, CT 06134-0308
(860) 509-7995
(860) 509-7910 (fax)

James C. Welch, R.N.
HIV/STD/AIDS
Delaware Division of Public Health
P.O. Box 637
Dover, DE 19903
(302) 739-4745
(302) 739-6617 (fax)

Vacant
Preventive Health Services Administration
Department of Public Health
800 9th Street, SW, 2nd Floor
Washington, DC 20024
(202) 645-5550
(202) 645-0454 (fax)

Landis Crockett, M.D., M.P.H.
Division Director, Office of Disease Control
Florida Department of Health
1317 Winewood Boulevard
Tallahassee, FL 32399-0700
(850) 921-2220
(850) 487-1521 (fax)

William C. Fields
Deputy Director, Division of Public Health
Georgia Department of Human Resources
7th Floor, Suite 300
2 Peachtree Street
Atlanta, GA 30303-3186
(404) 657-2700
(404) 657-2715 (fax)

Dennis Rodriquez
Department of Public Health and Social Services
Government of Guam
P.O. Box 2816
Agana, GU 96910
9-011 (671) 734-7101
9-011 (671) 734-5910 (fax)

Peter Whiticar
STD/HIV Prevention Program
Department of Health
3627 Kilauea Avenue, Room 304
Honolulu, HI 94816-2399
(808) 733-9010
(808) 733-9015 (fax)

Roger Perotto
Chief, Bureau of Clinical and Preventive Services
Department of Health and Welfare
450 West State Street, 4th Floor
Boise, ID 83720
(208) 334-0670
(208) 334-6581 (fax)

Charles Rabins, M.P.H.
Acting Chief, Division of Infectious Diseases
Illinois Department of Public Health
525 West Jefferson Street
Springfield , IL 62761
(217) 782-2747
(217) 524-5443 (fax)

Christine Kosmos
Administrative Director, Health Protection Division
Chicago Department of Health
333 South State Street, 2nd Floor
Chicago, IL 60604
(312) 747-9696
(312) 747-9420 (fax)
(313)

Michael Wallace, Director
Division of HIV/STD
Indiana Department of Health
2 North Meridian Street
P.O. Box 1964
Indianapolis, IN 46204
(317) 233-7867
(317) 233-7663 (fax)

John R. Kelly, Director
Division of Health Protection
Department of Public Health
Lucas State Office Building
Des Moines, IA 50319-0075
(515) 281-7785
(515) 242-6284 (fax)

Paula Marmet, M.A.
Bureau of Disease Control
Department of Health and Environment
Mills Building, Suite 605
109 SW 9th Street
Topeka, KS 66612-1271
(913) 296-0022
(913) 296-4197 (fax)

Clarkson T. Palmer, M.D., M.P.H.
Manager, Communicable Disease Branch
Division of Epidemiology
Kentucky Department of Health Services
275 East Main Street
Frankfort, KY 40621
(502) 543-3263
(502) 564-6533 (fax)

Thomas Farley, M.D., M.P.H.
Administrator, STD Control Program
Office of Public Health
Department of Health and Hospitals
325 Loyola Avenue
New Orleans, LA 70112
(504) 568-5005
(504) 568-5279 (fax)

Sally Lou Patterson
Acting Project Director, STD/HIV Program
Department of Human Services
State House, Station #11
Augusta, ME 04333
(207) 287-5551
(207) 287-6865 (fax)

Isamu Abraham, M.D.
Secretary of Health and Environmental Services
Mariana Islands Department of Public Health
  and Environmental Services
P.O. Box 409 CK
Saipan, MP 96950
(607) 234-8950
(607) 234-8930 (fax)

Donald F. Copelle
Secretary for Health and Environment
Republic of the Marshall Islands
P.O. Box 16
Majuro, MH 96960
9-011-(692) 625-3355
9-011-(692) 625-3432 (fax)

Rafiq Miazad, M.D., M.P.H.
Acting Chief, Division of STD
Department of Health and Mental Hygiene
3rd Floor, Room 307-B
201 West Preston Street
Baltimore, MD 21201
(410) 225-6688
(410) 333-5529 (fax)

David C. Rose, M.D., F.A.A.P.
Assistant Commissioner
Preventive Medicine and Epidemiology
Baltimore City Health Department
210 Guilford Avenue, 3rd Floor
Baltimore, MD 21202
(410) 396-4438
(410) 625-0688 (fax)

Paul Etkind
STD Control Program
Department of Public Health
305 South Street
Boston, MA 02130-3597
(617) 983-6941
(617) 983-6962 (fax)

David Johnson, M.D.,
Chief Executive and Medical Officer
Michigan Department of Community Health
3423 North Martin Luther King Jr. Boulevard
Lansing, MI 48909
(517) 335-8024
(517) 335-9476 (fax)

Eliuel K. Pretrick, M.O., M.P.H.
Department of Health Services
FSM National Government
Palikir Station, PS 70
P.O. Box PS 70
Pohnpei FM 96941
9-011 (691) 320-2619
9-011 (691) 320-5263 (fax)

Jill M. DeBoer, M.P.H., Manager
AIDS/STD Prevention Services Section
Minnesota Department of Health
717 Delaware Street, SE
P.O. Box 9441
Minneapolis, MN 55440-9441
(612) 623-5698
(612) 623-5739 (fax)

Robert Hotchkiss, M.D., Chief
Office of Community Health Services
Mississippi State Department of Health
2423 North State Street
P.O. Box 1700
Jackson, MS 39215-1700
(601) 960-7725
(601) 960-7948 (fax)

Pam Walker
Deputy Director, Division of Environment
Health and Communicable Disease Prevention
930 Wildwood
P.O. Box 570
Jefferson City, MO 65109
(573) 751-6080
(573) 751-6010 (fax)

Kathleen Martin
Communicable Disease Control and
  Prevention Bureau
Montana Department of Public Health
  and Human Services
Cogswell Building, Room C-305
Helena, MT 59620
(406) 444-4735
(406) 444-2920 (fax)

Christine M. Newlon, Director
Division of Disease Control
Department of Health
P.O. Box 95007
Lincoln, NE 68509-5007
(402) 471-2937
(402) 471-6426 (fax)

Yvonne Sylva
Administrator
Division of Health
Capitol Complex
505 East King Street, Room 201
Carson City, NV 89710
(702) 687-4740
(702) 687-4988 (fax)

David R. Ayotte, M.S.P.H.
STD/HIV Program
Bureau of Disease Control
6 Hazen Drive
Concord, NH 03301-6527
(603) 271-4502
(603) 271-4934 (fax)

Janet DeGraaf, M.P.A., Acting Director
Communicable Disease Control Service
New Jersey Department of Health
3635 Quakerbridge Road
P.O. Box 369
Trenton, NJ 08625-0369
(609) 588-7535
(609) 588-7431 (fax)

Donald Torres
HIV/AIDS/STD Prevention and Services
525 Camino De Los Marquez, Suite 1
Santa Fe, NM 87501
(505) 827-2389
(505) 827-2329 (fax)

F. Bruce Coles, D.O., Medical Director
Bureau of STD Control
New York State Department of Health
ESP Corning Tower, Room 1168
Albany, NY 12237
(518) 474-3598
(518) 474-3491 (fax)

Issac Weisfuse, M.D.
Assistant Commissioner
Bureau of STD Control
NYC Department of Health
125 Worth Street, Box 73
New York, NY 10013
(212) 788-4406
(212) 788-4431 (fax)

Evelyn B. Foust, M.P.H.
HIV/STD Prevention and Care Section
Department of Health and Human Services
P.O. Box 29601
Raleigh, NC 27626-0601
(919) 733-9490
(919) 733-1020 (fax)

Fred F. Heer
Division of Disease Control
North Dakota Department of Health
State Capitol Building
600 East Boulevard Avenue
Bismarck, ND 58505-0200
(701) 328-2378
(701) 328-1412 (fax)

William Ryan
Director of Health
Department of Health
246 North High Street
P.O. Box 118
Columbus, OH 43266-0588
(614) 466-2253
(614) 644-0085 (fax)

William R. Pierson
STD/HIV Service
Oklahoma State Department of Health
1000 N.E. 10th Street
Oklahoma City, OK 73117-1299
(405) 271-4636
(405) 271-7339 (fax)

Dave Fleming, M.D.
STD Program
Oregon Health Division
800 N.E. Oregon Street, Suite 730
Portland, OR 97232
(503) 731-4026
(503) 731-4082 (fax)

Anthony Pollai, M.D.
Director, Bureau of Health Services
Republic of Palau
P.O. Box 100
Koror, Palau PW 96940
9-011 (680) 488-2813
9-011 (680) 488-1211 (fax)

V. Diane Woods, R.N., M.S.N.
Bureau of Preventive Health Programs
Pennsylvania Department of Health
P.O. Box 90
Harrisburg, PA 17108
(717) 787-3981
(717) 783-5498 (fax)

Robert Levensen
Director, Division of Disease Control
Philadelphia Department of Public Health
500 South Broad Street
Philadelphia, PA 19146
(215) 685-6740
(215) 545-8362 (fax)

SylVetto Soto, M.D
PASET STD/HIV Prevention Section
Puerto Rico Department of Health
Central Medico, Building A, 2nd Floor
P.O. Box 70184
San Juan, PR 00936
(787) 274-5634
(787) 274-5523 (fax)

Paul Loberti Jr., M.P.H.
Division of Disease Control
Department of Health
Three Capitol Hill, Room 106
Providence, RI 02908-5097
(401) 277-2320
(401) 272-3771 (fax)

Lynda Kettinger, M.P.H.
South Carolina Department of Health
   and Environment Control
Mills/Jarrett Complex
1751 Calhoun Street
Columbia, SC 29201
(803) 737-4110
(803) 737-3979 (fax)

John N. Jones
Health, Medical and Laboratory Services
Department of Health
615 East 4th Street
Pierre, SD 57501
(605) 773-3737
(605) 773-5509 (fax)

Bill Moore, M.D.
Communicable Disease/STD
Tennessee Department of Health
Cordell Hull Building, 4th Floor
Nashville, TN 37247
(615) 532-8516
(615) 532-8478 (fax)

Vacant
Chief, Bureau of HIV and STD Prevention
Department of Health
1100 West 49th Street
Austin, TX 78756
(512) 490-2505
(512) 490-2544(fax)

Craig R. Nichols, M.P.A.
Bureau of Epidemiology
Department of Health
288 North 1460 West
P.O. Box 142870
Salt Lake City, UT 84114-2870
(801) 538-6191
(801) 538-9923 (fax)

Peter D. Galbraith, D.M.D., M.P.H.
Health Surveillance Division
Vermont Department of Health
108 Cherry Street
P.O. Box 70
Burlington, VT 05402
(802) 863-7225
(802) 865-7701 (fax)

Jose Poblete, M.D.
Commissioner of Health
Virgin Islands Department of Health
St. Thomas Hospital
48 Sugar Estate
St. Thomas, VI 00802
(809) 774-0117
(809) 777-4001 (fax)

Vacant
Office of Epidemiology
Virginia Department of Health
1500 East Main Street, Room 113
P.O. Box 2448
Richmond, VA 23218
(804) 786-6029
(804) 786-1076 (fax)

Larry Klopfenstein
Director, STD/TB Services
Department of Health
New Market Industrial Campus
7211 Cleanwater Lane, Building 14
Olympia, WA 98504-7842
(360) 236-3460
(360) 236-3470 (fax)

Loretta E. Haddy, M.S., M.A.
Surveillance and Disease Control
STD Program
West Virginia Department of Health
   and Human Services
1422 Washington Street, East
Charleston, WV 25301
(304) 558-2950
(304) 558-6335 (fax)

Jerald L. Young, M.P.H.
Chief, Communicable Disease Section
Department of Health and Family Services
1414 East Washington Avenue
Madison, WI 53703-3044
(608) 266-5819
(608) 266-2906 (fax)

Jimm Murray, Deputy Administrator
Branch of Preventive Medicine
Hathaway Building, 4th Floor
Cheyenne, WY 82002
(307) 777-6004
(307) 777-5402 (fax)

APPENDIX D

STD PREVENTION PARNERSHIP

The Centers for Disease Control and Prevention's National STD Prevention Partnership convenes more than 30 national organizations, including the National Conference of State Legislatures, which are concerned about the continuing spread of STDs, including HIV infection. The partnership began in 1992 with the mission to support and encourage partnerships among the private, voluntary and public sectors in developing and implementing plans to reduce the incidence and effects.

Frank Beadle de Palomo, M.A.
Academy for Educational Development
1255 23rd Street, N.W.
Washington, DC 20037
(202) 884-8700; (202) 884-8883; (202) 884-8929
(202) 884-8713 (fax)

Kent Klindera, HIV/AIDS Program Associate
Advocates for Youth
1025 Vermont Avenue, N.W., Suite 200
Washington, DC 20005
(202) 347-5700
(202) 347-2263 (fax)

Lisa Kaeser
Alan Guttmacher Institute
1120 Connecticut Avenue, N.W.
Washington, DC 20036
(202) 296-4012
(202) 223-5756 (fax)

Jacqueline Admire, M.S.P.H.
American Academy of Family Physicians
8880 Ward Parkway
Kansas City, MO 64114-2797
(816) 333-9700, Ext. 5500
(800) 274-2237, Ext. 5500
(816) 333-9855 (fax)

Ms. Laura Saul-Edwards
American Academy of Family Physicians
2021 Massachusetts Avenue, N.W.
Washington, DC 20036
(202) 232-9033
(202) 232-9044 (fax)

Carolyn Lopez, M.D.
Department of Family Practice
1900 W. Polk Street, 13th Floor
Chicago, IL 60612
(312) 633-8587
(312) 633-8454 (fax)

American Academy of Pediatrics
141 N.W. Point Boulevard
P.O. Box 927
Elk Grove Village, IL 60007-0927
(708) 228-5005
(708) 228-5027 (fax)

Alain Joffe, M.D., M.P.H.
Director of Adolescent Medicine
Johns Hopkins Hospital
600 N Wolfe Street, Park 307
Baltimore, MD 21287-2530
(410) 955-2910
(410) 955-4079 (fax)

Felicia Bloom, Project Director
Women's Health Initiatives
American Association of Health Plans
1129 20th Street, N.W., Suite 600
Washington, D.C. 20036
(202) 778-8471
(202) 778-3287

Janet Chapin, R.N., M.P.H., Associate Director
Division of Women's Health
American College of Obstetricians and Gynecologists
409 12th Street, S.W.
Washington, DC 20024-2188
(202) 638-5577; (202) 863-2579
(202) 484-3917 (fax)

Brandy Gress
American Indian Health Care Association
1999 Broadway, Suite 2530
Denver, CO 80202
(303) 295-3757
(303) 295-3390 (fax)

John Henning, Ph.D.
Department of STD and HIV
American Medical Association
515 North State Street
Chicago, IL 60610
(312) 464-4566
(312) 464-5841 (fax)

Peggy Veroneau
American Nurses Foundation
600 Maryland Avenue, S.W., Suite 100 West
Washington, DC 20024-2571
(202) 651-7068
(202) 651-7001 (fax)

Ann Burns, Associate Director of Education
American Pharmaceutical Association
2215 Constitution Avenue, N.W.
Washington, DC 20037
TEL: (202) 429-7581
FAX: (202) 783-2351

Catherine Stover
American Public Health Association
1015 15th Street, N.W.
Washington, DC 20005
(202) 789-5600
(202) 789-5661 (fax)

Joan Cates
American Social Health Association
P.O. Box 13827
Research Triangle Park, NC 27709
(919) 361-8417/8400
(919) 361-8425 (fax)

Johanna Chapin
Association of Reproductive Health Professionals
2401 Pennsylvania Avenue, N.W., Suite 350
Washington, DC 20037-1718
(202) 466-3825
(202) 466-3826 (fax)

Darcy Steinberg
Association of State and Territorial Health Officials
1275 K Street, N.W., Suite 800
Washington, DC 20005-4006
(202) 371-9090
(202) 371-9797 (fax)

Ms. Judy Lipshutz, M.P.H.
Communications and External Relations Office
Centers for Disease Control and Prevention
Division of STD Prevention
1600 Clifton Road, N.E., E02
Atlanta, GA 30333
(404) 639-8260
(404) 639-8608 (fax)

Cassandra A. Sparrow, Director
National Health Program
Congress of National Black Churches Inc., (CNBC)
1225 I Street, N.W., Suite 750
Washington, DC 20005-3914
(202) 371-1091
(202) 371-0908 (fax)

Bernice Humphrey, M.P.A.
Girls Incorporated
441 West Michigan Street
Indianapolis, IN 46202
(317) 634-7546
(317) 634-3024 (fax)

Berverly Wright, C.N.M., M.S.N., M.P.H.
Health Resources and Services Administration
c/o Division of Healthy Start
Maternal and Child Health Bureau
U.S. Department of Health and Human Services
5600 Fishers Lane, Room 11A-05
Rockville, MD 20857
(301) 443-8427
(301) 594-0186 (fax)

Rita Goodman
Health Resources and Services Administration
Bureau of Primary Health Care
Division of Community and Migrant Health
4350 East-West Highway, 7th Floor
Bethesda, MD 20814
(301) 594-4297
(301) 594-4997 (fax)

David M. Stevens, M.D.
HRSA/Bureau of Primary Health Care
Division of Community and Migrant Health
4350 East-West Highway, 7th Floor
Bethesda, MD 20814
(301) 594-4293; (301) 594-4297
(301) 594-4997 (fax)

Angela R. Powell, Deputy Chief
HRSA/Bureau of Health Resources Development
Division of HIV Services
5600 Fishers Lane, Room 7A-19
Rockville, MD 20857
(301) 443-9086
(301) 443-5271 (fax)

Laura Shelby, STD Director
Communicable Disease Epidemiology Branch
Indian Health Service
5300 Homestead Road, N.E.
Albuquerque, NM 87110
(505) 248-4395
(505) 248-4393 (fax)

Julie Scofield
National Alliance of State and Territorial
   AIDS Directors
444 North Capitol Street, N.W., Suite 706
Washington, DC 20001-1512
(202) 434-8090
(202) 434-8092 (fax)

Kenyon C. Burke, Ed.D, Consultant
ATTN: National Health Care Committee
National Association for the Advancement of
   Colored People
260 5th Avenue, 6th Floor
New York, NY 10001-6408
(973) 762-6725 (home)
(973) 762-4676 (business)
(973) 762-7844 (fax)

Tom Curtin, M.D.
Associate Vice President, Clinical Affairs
National Association of Community Health Centers
1330 New Hampshire Avenue, N.W., Suite 122
Washington, DC 20036
(616) 536-0379
(616) 536-0482 (fax)

Michael Meit, Research Associate
National Association of County and City
   Health Officials
440 First Street, N.W., Suite 500
Washington, DC 20001
(202) 783-5550
(202) 783-1583 (fax)

Ms. Susan J. Wysocki, R.N., President
National Association of Nurse Practitioners in
   Reproductive Health (NANPRH)
503 Capitol Court, N.E., Suite 300
Washington, DC 20002
(202) 543-9693
(202) 543-9858 (fax)

Chris Knutson, Board President
The Center for Health Training
400 Tower Building
1809 Seventh Avenue
Seattle, WA 98101-1316
(206) 447-9538
(206) 447-9539 (fax)

Elisa Luna
National Association of People with AIDS
1413 K Street, N.W., 7th Floor
Washington, DC 20005
(202) 898-0414, ext 108
(202) 898-0435 (fax)

Eliana Loveluck, Program Director
National Coalition of Hispanic Health and
   Human Services Organizations (COSSMHO)
1501 Sixteenth Street, N.W.
Washington, DC 20036-1401
(202) 387-5000
(202) 797-4353 (fax)

Charlie Rabins
National Coalition of STD Directors
Division of STD Control Section
Department of Public Health
515 West Jefferson
Springfield, IL 62761
(217) 782-2747
(217) 524-5443 (fax)

Lisa Speissegger
HIV, STD and Adolescent Health Project
National Conference of State Legislatures
1560 Broadway, Suite 700
Denver, CO 80202
(303) 830-2200
(303) 863-8003 (fax)

Kenyon C. Burke, Ed.D.
National Council of Churches
475 Riverside Drive
New York, NY 10115
(973) 762-4676
(973) 762-7844 (fax)

Miriam Torres
NCLR Center for Health Promotion
National Council of La Raza
1111 19th Street, N. W., Suite 1000
Washington, D.C. 20036
(202) 785-1670
(202) 785-0851 (fax)

Valerie Rochester, Director
HIV/STD Prevention Initiative
National Council of Negro Women
633 Pennsylvania Avenue, N.W.
Washington, DC 20004
(202)737-0120
(202) 737-0476 (fax)

Julia Mitchell
National Education Association Health
   Information Network
1201 16th Street, N.W., 5th Floor
Washington, DC 20036
(202) 822-7570; (202) 822-7723
(202) 822-7775 (fax)

Marilyn Keefe
National Family Planning and Reproductive
   Health Association
122 C Street, N.W., Suite 380
Washington, DC 20001-2109
(202) 628-3535
(202) 737-2690 (fax)

Marsha Hollomon
National Lesbian and Gay Health Association
1407 S Street, N.W.
Washington, DC 20009
(202) 939-7880
(202) 234-1467 (fax)

William E. Brown, M.D.
Assistant Professor OBGYN
National Medical Association
C/O Howard University Hospital
2041 Georgia Avenue, N.W.
Washington, DC 20068
(202) 865-4162
(202) 865-6922 (fax)

Gretchen Noll, Director
Safe Choices
National Network for Youth
1319 F Street, N.W., Suite 401
Washington, DC 20004
(202) 783-7949
(202) 783-7955 (fax)

Linda Fisher, M.D.
National STD/HIV Prevention/Training Center
  Network
C/O St. Louis County Department of Health
111 South Meramec Avenue
Clayton, MO 63105
(314) 854-6600
(314) 854-6435

Anne Hill, Director
Employment, Training, and Advocacy
National Urban League Inc.
500 East 62nd Street, 10th Floor
New York, NY 10021
(212) 310-9232
(212) 593-8250 (fax)

Cindy Pearson
Executive Director
National Women's Health Network
514 10th Street, N.E, #400
Washington, D.C. 20004
(202) 347-1140
(202) 347-1168 (fax)

Alvin Goldfarb, M.D.
Executive Director
North American Society for Pediatric and
  Adolescent Gynecology
1015 Chestnut Street, #1225
Philadelphia, PA 19107
(215) 955-6331
(215) 923-3474 (fax)

Susan B. Moskosky, M.S., R.N.C.
Director, Title X Training and Regional Activities
Office of Population Affairs
U.S. Department of Health and Human Services
East-West Towers, Suite 200 West
4350 East West Highway
Bethesda, MD 20814
(301) 594-4008
(301) 594-5980 (fax)

Leslie M. Hardy, Senior Policy Analyst
Division of Public Health Policy
Office of the Assistant Secretary for Planning
  and Evaluation
U.S. Department of Health and Human Services
Humphrey Building, Room 442E
200 Independence Avenue, SW
Washington, DC 20201
(202) 260-5156
(202) 690-6167 (fax)

John D. Siegfried, M.D., Associate Vice President
  Medical Affairs
Pharmaceutical Research and Manufacturers of
  America
1100 15th Street, N.W.
Washington, DC 20005
(202) 835-3545
(202) 835-3597 (fax)

Kara Anderson, R.N.C., B.A.
Director, Medical Affairs
Planned Parenthood Federation of America
810 7th Avenue, 12th Floor
New York, NY 10019
(212) 261-4700
(212) 261-6269

Chris Portelli
Sexuality Information and Education Council
  of the United States
130 West 42nd Street, 25th Floor
New York, NY 10036
(212) 819-9770, ext 305
(212) 819-9776 (fax)

Society for Adolescent Medicine
Suite 120
19401 East 40 Highway
Independence, MO 64055

Alain Joffe, M.D., M.P.H.
Director of Adolescent Medicine
Johns Hopkins Hospital
600 N. Wolfe Street, Park 307
Baltimore, MD 21287-2530
(410) 955-2910
(410) 955-4079 (fax)

Margaret Anderson, M.A.
Society for the Advancement of Women's
  Health Research
1828 L Street, N.W., Suite 625
Washington, DC 20036
(202) 223-8224
(202) 833-3472 (fax)

Adolfo Mata
Acting Associate Administrator for AIDS
Substance Abuse and Mental Health Services
  Administration
Parklawn Building; Room 12C-05
5600 Fishers Lane
Rockville, MD 20857
301-443-7015
301-443-7590 (fax)

Crystal Swann
United States Conference of Mayors
1620 Eye Street, N.W.
Washington, DC 20006
(202) 293-7330
(202) 887-0652 (fax)

Carmelita Gallo
Director, Community Resources
YMCA of the U.S.A.
101 North Wacker Drive, Suite 1400
Chicago, IL 60606
(800) 872-9622; (312) 269-0511
(312) 977-9063 (fax)

Alpha Alexander, Ph.D.
Director of Health Promotion and Sports
YWCA of the U.S.A.
350 Fifth Ave., Suite 301
New York, NY 10118
(212) 273-7960
(212) 273-7969 (fax)

NOTES

1. Centers for Disease Control and Prevention, "Summary of Notifiable Diseases, United States 1996," *Morbidity and Mortality Weekly Report* 45, no. 53, (1997).

2. E. Ambruster-Morales, L.M. Ioshimoto, E. Leao, and M. Zugaib, "Detection of Human Papillomavirus Deoxyribonucleic Acid Sequences in Amniotic Fluid During Different Periods of Pregnancy," *American Journal of Obstetrics and Gynecology* 169, (1993): 1074-5.

3. Centers for Disease Control and Prevention, "HIV Prevention Through Early Detection and Treatment of Other Sexually Transmitted Diseases—United States: Recommendations of the Advisory Committee for HIV and STD Prevention," *Morbidity and Mortality Weekly Report* 47, no. RR-12, (July 31, 1998):2.

4. H. Grosskurth, et al., "Impact of Improved Treatment of Sexually Transmitted Diseases on HIV Infection in Rural Tanzania: Randomized Controlled Trial," *Lancet* 346 (1995): 530-36.

5. William Cates, Jr., "Epidemiology and Control of Sexually Transmitted Diseases in Adolescents," *AIDS and Other Sexually Transmitted Diseases*, eds. M. Schydlower and M.A. Shager, (Philadelphia: Hanly & Belfus Inc., 1990), 409-27.

6. Thomas R. Eng and William T. Butler, eds. *The Hidden Epidemic: Confronting Sexually Transmitted Diseases* (Washington, D.C.: National Academy Press, 1997): 10.

7. American Social Health Association, "Teenagers know more than adults about STDs, but knowledge among both groups is low." *STD News* (Research Triangle Park: ASHA, Winter 1996): 1-5.

8. Centers for Disease Control and Prevention. *Sexually Transmitted Disease Surveillance, 1996* (Atlanta: CDC, 1997).

9. J. Paavonen, L.A. Koutsky, and N. Kiviat, "Cervical Neoplasia and Other STD-Related Genital and Anal Neoplasias," *Sexually Transmitted Diseases*, 2nd K.K. Holmes et al., eds. (New York: McGraw-Hill Inc., 1990): 561-92.

10. S.H. Ebrahim, T.A. Perterman, A.A. Zaidi, M.L. Kamb, "Mortality Related to Sexually Transmitted Diseases in Women, U.S., 1973 – 1992" (Eleventh Meeting of the International Society for STD Research, August 27-30, 1995, New Orleans [abstract no. 343]).

11. AIDS Information Exchange, "HIV and Other STDs: How Do They Fit Together?"

12. The Henry J. Kaiser Family Foundation, Kaiser Family Foundation/*Glamour* National Survey—"Talking About STDs with Health Professionals: Women's Experiences, Summary of Findings" (Menlo Park, Calif., 1997).

13. Centers for Disease Control and Prevention, "STDs and Pregnancy" (Atlanta: CDC, October 1997).

14. Ibid.

15. Ibid.

16. Ibid.

17. Centers for Disease Control and Prevention, "Recommendations for Human Immunodeficiency Virus Counseling and Voluntary Testing for Pregnant Women." *Morbidity and Mortality Weekly Report* 44, no. RR-7, (1995): ii.

18. K.E. Toomey, J.S. Moran, M.P. Raffety, G.A. Beckett, "Epidemiological Considerations of Sexually Transmitted Diseases in Underserved Populations." *Infectious Disease Clinics of North America* 7, (1993): 739-52.

19. Centers for Disease Control and Prevention. *Sexually Transmitted Disease Surveillance, 1996* (Atlanta: CDC, 1997).

20. Ibid.

21. Thomas R. Eng and William T. Butler, eds. *The Hidden Epidemic: Confronting Sexually Transmitted Diseases* (Washington, D.C.: National Academy Press, 1997) **?.**

22. Ibid., 58.

23. Ibid., 58.

24. Ibid., 58.

25. A.E. Washington and P. Katz, "Cost of and Payment Source for Pelvic Inflammatory Disease: Trends and Projections, 1983 through 2000" *Journal of the American Medical Association* 266, (1991): 2565-9.

26. Thomas R. Eng and William T. Butler, eds. *The Hidden Epidemic: Confronting Sexually Transmitted Diseases* (Washington, D.C.: National Academy Press, 1997): 175.

27. Ibid., 175-176.

28. Ibid., 177.

29. C.L. Celum et al., "Where Would Clients Seek Care for STD Services Under Health Care Reform? Results of an STD Client Survey from Five Clinics" (Eleventh Meeting of the International Society for STD Research, August 27-30, 1995, New Orleans [abstract no. 101]).

30. Thomas R. Eng and William T. Butler, eds. *The Hidden Epidemic: Confronting Sexually Transmitted Diseases* (Washington, D.C.: National Academy Press, 1997): 178.

31. Ibid., 185-186.

32. Ibid., 187-188.

33. M. Guiden, "School-Based Health Centers and Managed Care" *State Legislative Report* 23 (Denver: National Conference of State Legislatures, April 1998), 11.

34. Thomas R. Eng and William T. Butler, eds. *The Hidden Epidemic: Confronting Sexually Transmitted Diseases* (Washington, D.C.: National Academy Press, 1997): 187.

35. R. Brackbill, (Unpublished Data, 1997).

36. Institute of Medicine, *The Future of Public Health* (Washington, D.C.: National Academy Press, 1988).

37. A.M. Brandt, *No Magic Bullet: A Social History of Venereal Disease in the United States Since 1880* (New York: Oxford University Press, 1987).

38. Centers for Disease Control and Prevention, *Strategic Plan for the Division of STD Prevention and FY97 Principal Priorities by Core Function and Branch/Office with Lead or Co-Lead Responsibility* (Atlanta: CDC, October 1996).

39. Thomas R. Eng and William T. Butler, eds. *The Hidden Epidemic: Confronting Sexually Transmitted Diseases* (Washington, D.C.: National Academy Press, 1997): 208.

40. Centers for Disease Control and Prevention. *Sexually Transmitted Disease Surveillance, 1996* (Atlanta: CDC, 1997).

41. American Social Health Association, *ASHA Action* (Research Triangle Park: ASHA, April 1997).

42. Medical Institute for Sexual Health, *Sexual Health Update* (Austin: MISH, Spring 1998).

43. D. Kirby et al., "School-Based Programs to Reduce Sexual Risk Behaviors: A Review of Effectiveness," *Public Health Reports* 109, no. 3 (May – June 1994).

44. D.A. Cohen et al., "A School-Based Chlamydia Control Program Using DNA Amplification Technology," *Pediatrics* 101, no. 1 (1998): e1 – 10.

45. Eng, Thomas R. Butler, William, T., eds. *The Hidden Epidemic: Confronting Sexually Transmitted Diseases* (Washington, D.C.: National Academy Press, 1997): 195.

46. Centers for Disease Control and Prevention, *CDC Update* (Atlanta: CDC, August 1998).

47. Center for Health Training, "Region X Infertility Project" (Seattle: CFHT, 1997).

48. Centers for Disease Control and Prevention, *CDC Update* (Atlanta: CDC, August 1998).

49. Ibid.

50. Eng, Thomas R. and Butler, William T., eds. *The Hidden Epidemic: Confronting Sexually Transmitted Diseases* (Washington, D.C.: National Academy Press, 1997): 3.

51. Centers for Disease Control and Prevention. "1998 Guidelines for Treatment of Sexually Transmitted Diseases," Morbidity *and Mortality Weekly Report* 47, no. RR-1, (1998): 1.

52. L.O. Gostin et al., *Improving State Law to Prevent and Treat Infectious Disease* (New York: Milbank Memorial Fund, 1998).

53. Ibid.

54. Ibid.

55. Centers for Disease Control and Prevention, *Focus on STD Prevention* (Atlanta: CDC, November 1996).